Stress

Philip Cowell is an author, copywriter and poet. He has an eclectic mindfulness background and has participated in the Mindfulness-Based Stress Reduction course and other mindfulness-related training, including Focusing, Hakomi, Feldenkrais, Sacred Clown, and Courage and Renewal. He teaches creative writing in different settings and integrates mindfulness into his workshops. <www.philipcowell.co.uk>

Lorraine Millard has been a UKCP registered psychotherapist and supervisor for many years. She has also been a trainer and consultant for counselling and psychotherapy training since the 1990s. She is a mindfulness teacher and integrates mindfulness into all of her work with groups and individuals. <www.lorrainemillard.com>

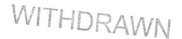

Sheldon Mindfulness

Selected titles

A full list of titles is available from Sheldon Press,
36 Causton Street, London SW1P 4ST and on our website at
www.sheldonpress.co.uk

Anxiety and Depression
Dr Cheryl Rezek

Compassion
Caroline Latham

Keeping a Journal
Philip Cowell

Quit Smoking
Dr Cheryl Rezek

Stress
Philip Cowell and Lorraine Millard

Sheldon Mindfulness

Stress

PHILIP COWELL
and
LORRAINE MILLARD

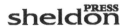
sheldon **PRESS**

First published in Great Britain in 2016

Sheldon Press
36 Causton Street
London SW1P 4ST
www.sheldonpress.co.uk

British Library Cataloguing-in-Publication Data
A catalogue record for this book is available from the British Library

ISBN 978–1–84709–376–9
eBook ISBN 978–1–84709–377–6

Typeset by Fakenham Prepress Solutions, Fakenham, Norfolk NR21 8NN
First printed in Great Britain by Ashford Colour Press
Subsequently digitally reprinted in Great Britain

eBook by Fakenham Prepress Solutions, Fakenham, Norfolk NR21 8NN

Produced on paper from sustainable forests

Dedicated to
mindfulness teachers and students
and the loveliness
of lifelong learning

Contents

Acknowledgements   viii

1   There's something lovely about you (no matter how
        stressed out you are)   1
2   This is your big moment: a bit more on mindfulness   16
3   What stress is and why it's one of the most interesting
        things about you   39
4   From stressfulness to mindfulness – going deeper   56
5   Loving every moment   75

Further reading   83

Acknowledgements

Thank you to Fiona Marshall at Sheldon Press for inviting us to write this book. You've been so supportive throughout – and patient and very generous.

This is a book that very much champions the teacher–student relationship, and so we have to acknowledge greatly the teachers who have helped us so much. Thank you especially to Jon Kabat-Zinn, Cindy Cooper and Sarah Silverton.

Thank you from Lorraine to Scott, Mack and Sara, and Sarah S. for patient and endless support and for my most constant role models in mindfulness, Libby and Reg, the labradors.

Given family is where we often learn the most about stress, thank you in a really good way from Philip to my mum and dad, Sue and Dave, to my middle brother Anthony, his wife Michelle and their gorgeous kids, Jake and Isobel, and to my older brother Ben, his wife Jules and their fantastic boys, Reuben and Toby. As the poet Michael Donaghy said, 'My people were magicians.'

Sheldon Mindfulness

Stress

1

There's something lovely about you (no matter how stressed out you are)

If you've ever said, 'I'm so stressed!' this book is for you

If you've never said it, but have thought it, it's also for you. No matter what kind of stress you've experienced, given there are many different kinds, this book is for you. Whatever stress is, it's something worth thinking about; it's worth taking the time to double check how we feel about it and relate to it.

And if you're particularly interested in how you might be able to bring mindfulness – the practice of simply being in the moment – to your stress, then this book is most definitely for you. It's for you whether you know something about mindfulness or not. But wait, let's slow down. We're getting ahead of ourselves. Let's not get stressed now.

To begin at the beginning (as someone famous once said)

Before we get into wondering what mindfulness is – assuming you've picked this book up because you're at least curious about it – I would like you to take a moment to just stop and be with yourself.

In a moment, after you've read these few sentences, stop what you're doing and just be. It's harder than you might think! You might be in a bookshop, or one of those places we used to call libraries, or you might be at home having downloaded this to your e-reader, or at work on your lunch break, on a crowded train with your noisy kids, or on the bus heading somewhere nice (or not nice).

Pause, look and listen to the things around you

Wherever and whoever you are, just take this moment to stop and be; bringing attention to yourself, noticing yourself in this moment. Take yourself by the hand and guide yourself round this moment. You might notice things like objects, sounds, feelings; there might be expectations, other people, or even just your plain old breathing. Notice all of them. Acknowledge them without trying to get rid of them or following them. Simply let them be, and let yourself be with them. Take a minute or two. Literally, enjoy yourself.

This is mindfulness

Holding onto yourself in this way – letting things be as they are, letting them come and go – is what we call mindfulness. That's as easy and as difficult as it gets.

Knowing that, I would like you now to read this next sentence to yourself – either out loud, if you can, or in your head if you can't. So get back to that place you were just in – that place of noticing yourself, your body's sensations, your breathing, your quietness, with your eyes shut if that works for you; and, when you're ready, read this sentence out loud, or in your head:

There's something lovely about me.

Give yourself some time with that. This is an unusual thing to do, of course, let's recognize that right away, particularly if you've said it out loud on a train. But even before we wonder how it feels, let's try it again. So, sitting or standing or walking along quietly, say out loud – either in your head, or to the world:

There's something lovely about me.

How was it that second time? You don't have to wonder what it is that's lovely about you. You might not even feel it's true. It could sound like I'm trying to flatter you (I'm not). You might have experienced some judging – something like 'This is a silly thing to do' – but let's not worry too much about our judgements.

Try again, this time taking extra notice of how you're breathing

Without changing your breathing, notice yourself breathing in and breathing out; even noticing, if you can, the gap in between. Do that and have one more go at this sentence, reading it either aloud or in your head (you could try both, observing any differences):

There's something lovely about me.

Did it feel OK to say it? Did you believe yourself? I wonder if it led to any thoughts or feelings that were compelling? I wonder, were they strong enough to take you off on a tangent, even off onto another story? Were you up for thinking – or feeling – that there is something lovely about you? Without labouring the point, I would like to suggest that there is indeed something lovely about you – whoever you are, wherever you are – and that I know so without even having to know who you are. You're just lovely, you are.

We might call the lovely thing about you your mindfulness

Your mindfulness is your aliveness. Your mindfulness – your aliveness – is your ability and capability to live in the present, ongoing moment, without judging yourself or the things happening around you; noticing simple things like your breath, or sounds. We might even throw in a smidgen of kindness too – mindfulness is a practice that involves being kind to yourself and, potentially, to others.

Listen to some music you like, and breathe

Throughout this book, we'll have some practical exercises for you to try. They're aimed at everybody, no matter how experienced or otherwise you are at mindfulness. This one's simple:

Put on some music you really like listening to. Whatever you fancy is great. It can be gentle classical music or the loudest heavy metal. For a few minutes, just listen to the music, to the sounds you hear and the sounds between sounds, and pay attention to the words, the music, the rhythms, the melody, the feelings behind the music. Notice your own breathing in and out as you listen. Notice the music coming to an end and then notice the silence after the music, all the time bringing some gentle awareness to your breathing.

Your mindfulness is a lot of things, but we can start with that. It's your ability to be you, plain and simple, in the moment, without distraction or judgement and with plenty of kindness. It's your ability not only to *not* criticize yourself, but to turn up to each moment in this ongoing present you find yourself in – called the present because it is, famously, very much a gift.

Your mindfulness is about you turning up and being aware of as much as possible of what is happening in your field of awareness, not following any particular thing as such, just letting all the things be. With your mindfulness, you're not following the sounds of the cars going by outside, you're just letting them be. You're not following the inner monologue about why you're so stressed, you're just letting it be. If you're elated – the happiest you've been for a while – your mindfulness whispers, 'This moment, like the stressful ones, will pass.' So, here too, you can find the stillness that runs through your life, like a thread through everything.

The reason there's something lovely about you has everything to do with you taking your life into your own hands. You're breathing and being you. That's an exceptional story to tell. Maybe you're coming back to yourself after you've been away. Maybe you're really good at being you (in which case, congratulations!). Maybe this is the hardest work on the planet and the minute you sit still with yourself your heart breaks open. Whatever condition you are in, if condition is an OK word to say here, there's something lovely about you: you've woken up to yourself, to what's already here, and you've done it in the nick of time.

And if you've come to this book because of stress, brilliant!

Stress is a great reason to want to become more mindful. The authors of this book have certainly held hands with their stresses and strains on their own paths to mindfulness. And if you've come to this book because you're stressed, or at least because you're interested in your relationship with stress, then even more brilliant. The good news is, the solution to your stress is already here. It's right under your nose: literally.

There are a few myths about stress that we'll be looking at

One myth about stress is that you need to be stressed to experience it. In a paradoxical way, it really helps, in fact, not to be stressed, in order that you can experience your stress. We'll be talking more about this.

Another myth is that stress exists in the first place. But does it? Or at least, what are we talking about when we talk about stress?

Even if stress does exist, what can mindfulness do about it? And conversely, what can stress do about your mindfulness? It might be a case of redescribing our stress and our relationship with it – through mindfulness – rather than eradicating stress altogether. Let's keep all these options in tow.

These are the key questions for this book and I hope you like the sound of them

Unlike classic self-help books, we're not going to claim we can solve your problems (actually, plenty of classic books don't claim that either). Truly, mindfulness isn't a cure-all. But mindfulness certainly can help you work on your relationship with stress, and that's a big enough start for now. In fact, rather than being a self-help book, we think of this as a Help-Yourself-to-Yourself book. So this book you have in your hands is saying something like: 'Here's mindfulness; help yourself to it.'

Give yourself a little half-smile the next time you have a free moment

Perhaps you're wandering along a riverbank, or in a shopping aisle, or watching the news, or writing a to-do list, or in a cave heading under-ground. Whatever you are doing, there will be a free moment at some point in amongst the busyness. In that free moment, inhale and exhale quietly three times without speaking or counting or changing the rate at which you breathe. Give yourself a little half-smile to acknowledge you've opened this space for yourself in amongst the rocks of your life. Be gentle with yourself. Even if you can't focus on the three in- and out-breaths, just allow what wants to happen to happen. You've been breathing your entire life; it's just that now you're coming afresh towards your secret breathing self. Breathing freshly in this way, knowing you are breathing, is mindfulness.

There's nothing mysterious about this

Mindfulness is just about being in the present moment, with all that it holds, and accepting that present moment for what it is, no matter what it is.

Mindfulness has a wonderful history. As you breathe in now, intentionally, bringing awareness to your act of breathing in and breathing out, noticing the pause between, you are connecting with over 2,500 years of breath-bodies breathing and knowing they are breathing. This knowing is called awareness. People have been sitting quietly in rooms for millennia, noticing their breathing.

Now's your time

Why? Because the benefits are exponential; because neuroscience and psychology are telling us great things about mindfulness and other embodied self-awareness practices; because through mindfulness come compassion, resilience and an all-encompassing kindness towards yourself and others around you; because, regardless of needing any proof whatsoever, you are alive and, somehow, ignoring that fact does you, and all of us, an injustice.

Breath and body are our best friends

In secular mindfulness, as it has been taught by pioneer teachers like Jon Kabat-Zinn, we learn to shift from the domain of doing to the domain of being. The frantic, frenzied running around and 'getting things done' becomes a gentle, quiet ambling back and forth. We learn to slow our bodies down and observe our minds and perceptions in a kind, calm and accepting way. We let thoughts come and go, we observe them; always we gently guide ourselves back to the breath and the body.

We're not the White Rabbit in Alice in Wonderland

We don't rush down the rabbit hole after our thoughts. We just look at them, greet them, identify or label them (making them clearer, and therefore making it clearer to ourselves not to follow them), and then let them go. In this moment, we return to our position – our sitting or standing – and we continue to focus on the breath and our contact with the earth. Our breath and our bodies are our best friends in mindfulness.

Breathing's the thing

Have you noticed your breath as you've been reading the last few pages? If not, don't worry, your body was probably doing the breathing for you. Breathing is one of the most beautiful, simple things we know. It's the bedrock of life. The breath of life is the stuff of life. Even the word 'animal' literally means 'have breath'. Think about it: you breathe from the moment you're born right through to the moment you die. And sure, I'm being simplistic here – there may be moments when machines have to do the breathing for you – but you get the point. Your breath is a thread that runs through you and your entire life. How you notice your breath right now is how you live your entire life.

Philip remembers the moment he realized he was a breathing being

I can recall it vividly to this day. It was during the news coverage surrounding the Hillsborough football disaster in April 1989 (I was eight) when 96 people were crushed to death and 766 people were injured. Mum was at the ironing board and Dad, who had been doing chores in town, came rushing into the room to tell us to put the TV on. I think it was during one of the news items about the disaster that I realized I was breathing (I can even remember where I sat on our floral settee). So I remember the first moment I realized I was breathing. This was then followed by panic, because I thought I had to keep remembering to breathe in order *to* breathe. I had the eight-year-old thought of 'What if I forget to breathe?' Of course, I then spent years forgetting to breathe, and 26 years later I'm here to tell the tale.

I look back now and of course I can see why. The news was full of the awful tragedy – people suffocating to death in the crush of the crowds – and there I was, sitting in the luxury of breathing, and noticing I was doing so. What I don't remember is then realizing – as

I must have done – that I didn't in fact need to remember to breathe; that our bodies breathe for us.

So the point about your breathing is that it is both automatic and non-automatic

Our bodies can do it with all awareness and consciousness, and they can also do it without even realizing or noticing. Freudian psycho-analysts think about the conscious and the unconscious, and hold that you only have access to the unconscious through dreams and Freudian slips of the tongue. Mindfulness practitioners don't have to think about things in those terms (they might, personally, but it's not part of mindfulness); instead they see things in terms of Things We're Aware Of In This Moment and Things We're Not Aware Of In This Moment. And it's those latter bits – the stuff of what we might call the automatic pilot – that we'll encounter a lot during our exploration of mindfulness.

Make yourself a mindful pot of tea

Mindfulness is there for you throughout your life, even – and especially – in the little moments, like making a pot of tea for you and a friend, or even – and especially – just for yourself.

Fill the kettle with kind awareness. How much water will you really need? Place the cups on the side with gentleness and reverence to gravity. Place the tea bags or leaves in the pot, knowing that when you do this, you are really doing it. When you switch the kettle on, really feel your finger press the switch. As you wait for the water to boil, stand upright and tall, as best you can, with ease, with the dignity of a mountain, and just breathe in. You may be aware of thoughts like, 'But I must go and speak to my friend', or 'I must get ready to pour the boiling water into the pot'. Let the thoughts be and just stand in the dignity of your present moment. Gently, when the kettle has boiled, pour the water into the teapot as if this is the first time you have ever done it. Pour with wonder. Let the steam stand for your amazement.

Even when we make a pot of tea, we can attend to the present moment in its fullness.

Invite your automatic pilot in for a cup of tea

How in touch with your body are you in this moment? Mindfulness is about bringing awareness to all aspects of your lived experience, including – and especially – to your body, which can often be found in automatic pilot mode. Automatic pilot is essential, of course; we can't be aware of everything all the time – or perhaps we can, but that might be a way off for even the most monkish of us.

The key here is to befriend your automatic pilot, sit up front with him or her in the cockpit of your life, and invite kind curiosity to the biplane of your body–mind. With mindfulness, you can show your automatic pilot that there is so much more to this flying and living malarky than just pressing some buttons and kicking back with a newspaper and a doughnut. (Apologies to actual pilots everywhere; I know you don't do that.)

To extend the metaphor (mindfulness does love a metaphor), you can invite your pilot to take the controls once more, unclick the automatic pilot button, and begin again to steer your life consciously and with beautiful mindfulness. Your pilot, now a conscious pilot, sees new things, lives more deeply, experiences the airscape on his or her skin, observes thoughts for what they are – simply thoughts – with you in the front seat, aware of all that is taking place. Rather than dwelling on past events or conjuring up future plans, your conscious pilot steers your life into open skies and existence through present, moment-to-moment attention, on purpose and without recourse to judgement.

According to Jon Kabat-Zinn, there are seven foundational attitudes to mindfulness

Crucial to mindfulness are the attitudes at the practice's foundation. The attitudes are words of honour – very familiar words from everyday language that are given a little more importance. The foundational attitudes – or important words – are:

- non-judging
- patience
- beginner's mind
- trust
- non-striving
- accepting
- letting go.

Like the stars and planets, they're all interconnected, so working on one attitude feeds all of the others. Let's look at each one in turn, they're each special in their own way.

Non-judging This means being able to allow thoughts to come, or sounds or your breathing, without judging them. With mindfulness, we don't judge thoughts like we do in everyday life. In fact, though we're hugely grateful to thinking and all it gives us, with mindfulness we try to get away from the thinking part of ourselves. Mindfulness involves stepping back in kindness from the chatter of thoughts and judgements in your head and allowing yourself to just be with them as you fall fully into your body. We sit on the banks and watch our thoughts pass us by as beautifully and naturally as a river. And of course if we start judging our thoughts, which is as natural as a river, rather than beating ourselves up for doing so, we observe the judging with kindness, and bring our attention gladly back to the interested, noticing mode (as opposed to the involved, swept-up one). The key with mindfulness is awareness, so that even if we 'break the rules' of mindfulness, we can still use our flouting of those rules as an opportunity to explore lived experience from all angles.

Patience This practice won't come overnight. It takes time. Mindfulness is like any art form in that way. Patience is the wisdom that kindness and slowing down, and not trying to push or get to the next moment, reveal so much more. There is so much going on in each single moment – tensions in the body, pressure through contact with the floor, the background hum of thinking and judging, the emerging of a felt sense of here and now – that if we can slow down and be patient for just one of those moments, we're doing really good work.

Beginner's mind Can we come to each moment with fresh new eyes, without bringing any assumptions from our past experience, or expectations about our future experience? A central tenet of mindfulness is **beginner's mind**. We could simply define beginner's mind as *looking afresh at the world each time*. How often do we see the same things in our daily lives, attend the same rituals (travelling to work, meeting the same people)? We could easily assume we know these people, the things we see. But how well do we really know them? What's new inside the same old same old? By practising mindfulness, we start again (or even start to start again); we bring freshness and newness to our experience and our experience *of* experience. However you find yourself in this moment, reading this page (which looks so similar to all those other pages), can you bring beginner's mind to your inner and outer experience of Page?

Trust Mindfulness practice gets tough, and when the going gets tough, trust in the going. As you sit, or stand, or lie down, you trust in the process. You trust in a process that is ancient, and deep, and connects you to thousands of people over the years who have responded to their life stresses and strains by slowing down and equipping themselves with their very own stillness. Trust, when you think about it, is beautiful.

Non-striving We're not trying to get anywhere, or to be anything other than who we are in the magnificence of this moment. With mindfulness, we don't strive to get that job interview or finish changing the beds so we can watch telly. We experience the fullness of how it feels to apply for a job or how the bed sheets feel ballooning out and now down as we change the bed in this beautiful moment. When we sit, or stand, or walk mindfully, we aren't trying to get anywhere. There is nowhere to get to, we are already here. And stress, *our* stress, is here too. That's why it potentially makes us retreat into our stressfulness. So we don't strive to get anywhere with our stress. We simply let it be. We let the stress be and it lets us be.

Acceptance However we are in this moment, we attend to it like our own inner butler. And in doing so we accept ourselves a little more. By turning up to this moment, we accept the moment – and ourselves in it – for what it is. Yes please, Jeeves, drive right up to the present moment. With mindfulness, we accept ourselves, and we do so in a radical way. Radically accepting ourselves means turning up to this moment. We are beautiful, we are ugly, we are carefree, we are stressed. Our mindfulness of stress practice helps us accept ourselves, and others around us, better.

Letting go We aren't clingy at all, when it comes to mindfulness. We aren't trying to keep things as they are; we let things go, and we notice our relationship with that act of letting go. With mindfulness, we practise letting go, and that includes letting go of our stress.

Wash the dishes mindfully

When it comes to clearing up the dishes after a meal, we can attend to them in an annoyed, stressful manner and say things like, 'Oh, I've got to do this again!' Or we can bring mindfulness to the encounter, and beginner-washerupper's mind, and say, 'Oh, I *get* to do this again.'

Following your breath, allow the soap suds to cover your hands and wrists, feel plate and fork and glass against your increasingly soft skin.

Bring slowness to your doing, so that you're working in a being kind of way. Being with washing up in this moment.

It's easier to write about that than to do it, and don't worry – there are plenty of times the authors of this book aren't mindful when doing the dishes. Oh, but the difference it makes!

A quick note on the authors

Before we go any further, let's introduce ourselves. We are friends who met on an eight-week mindfulness course. We didn't know each other before the course; we became friends very much as a result of mindfulness and the wonder it brings. Lorraine was the teacher (she's trained by the great mindfulness folk at Bangor University) and Philip was one of her students.

We write this book in the spirit of lifelong learning with which we both came to mindfulness in the first place. Though one of us is the teacher and one the student, we are both teachers and students to each other; and life, of course, is the ultimate teacher of mindfulness, and we are all its students. In fact, more than anything – more than an aid to rest and relaxation, more than a cure-all for life's woes (which of course it is not) – mindfulness is a living form of self-led lifelong learning. To learn the skills and receive the benefits of mindfulness is to engage in an ongoing enquiry into how to live a full and fascinating life. For that reason, we have enjoyed writing this book together as a kind of ode to teachers and students everywhere, and we have loved the excuse it has fostered to spend some extra time together.

Throughout the book, we refer to things that are useful to us, and personal to us, and so we sometimes start our sentences with 'I . . .' and sometimes with 'We . . .' We try to make it clear who is speaking if there is an 'I', but we're also not too worried if it's not so clear, and we hope you won't worry either. Whether it's an 'I' or a 'We', we're conveying simple truths that are hopefully useful to everyone; so it doesn't exactly matter *who* experienced them. We/I hope that's OK with you.

A quick note about you

Thank you for being here, first of all. We've been expecting you. We really are grateful that you chose our book – for now – out of the many that are available, as the one to read. Of course, we'd recommend plenty of the others – and there's a list of suggested reading at the end of this book to help you continue your investigations.

You might be coming to this book because you've got an interest in your own stress. Do bring your own stress to the party. We can only work on the material you bring. Though we will – in the nature of the beast – be talking about things not directly relevant to your specific life, do always relate our words to your own words. And our most important advice to you (though thankfully this book doesn't have much advice in it) is: do try and take part in one of the many eight-week mindfulness courses available, either in person, over the telephone or online. Again, details of those are available at the end of the book.

2

This is your big moment: a bit more on mindfulness

This is your big moment: this one, right now

This is the moment you can turn up and decide to reclaim your life as your own. If you've come to this book because you're stressed – or interested in your stress – and want to find another way to live your life, welcome; come in, both of you (your stress included).

Come in with your stress, take your shoes off if you wish, and sit down. Sit down here in the middle of your life, in the middle of your stress, and just be.

Sitting down quietly in amongst the hum and the drum of stress is exactly what mindfulness is all about. So this is your big moment. This one. Right now.

There is so much written about mindfulness

So much has been written about mindfulness, it's difficult to know where to start. We could easily get stressed about that. Hopefully you'll bear with us. And regardless of where we start, and how much is out there already, you're here, we're here, and we've got a wonderful job to do together: to discover what mindfulness is in as clear and simple a way as possible, and then see how it can help with our responses to stress.

Practise sitting meditation

Believe it or not, whoever you are, this is the middle of your life. When you attend to yourself with mindfulness, you find yourself right in the middle of things. This moment is here, right now, right here.

So take this moment to sit, plain and simple. Sit on a chair, or on a cushion on the floor, or on the sofa ... simply sit. Notice your breathing and notice you're breathing. If you like, count each in- and out-breath up to ten, so that the first in-breath is one, the first out-breath is one; the second in-breath is two, the second out-breath is two; and so on. If your mind wanders, which it inevitably will, you might forget which number you've reached. No worries. Just start counting again from one. Then, when you have got to ten, simply breathe and sit in the same way without counting. Notice your contact with the floor, your feet in cahoots with carpet or wooden panel, your buttocks on cushion or chair, your entire body pulling heartwards towards the centre of the earth. Well done. You're doing some fantastic sitting. Stay here for as long as feels right in this moment.

This is the heart of sitting meditation, a key mindfulness position, or dignity – the others are standing, lying down and walking – which we will return to lots. Practise sitting every day in this way, if you can, for however long feels good for you.

So what is mindfulness again?

'Mindfulness means paying attention in a particular way, on purpose, in the present moment, and non-judgmentally.' The creator of the original eight-week Mindfulness-Based Stress Reduction course, Jon Kabat-Zinn, wrote those words. Have another quick read of them.

Mindfulness means paying attention in a particular way:

- on purpose,

- in the present moment
- and non-judgementally.

Mindfulness, then, is about being really aware of your experience in this moment

Let's stress (in a non-stressful way) that mindfulness is about being *really* aware of your experiences as you are experiencing them, without judgement. No 'I shouldn't be feeling that', no 'I'm too old, too fat', no 'I'm a bad breather', no 'I can't do it'. And it's *all* you are experiencing that you're bringing your mindfulness to: all the sensations, the senses, the inside, the outside; all with a generous sprinkling of kindness to yourself. Too much to ask? In the classic formulation (you'll hear this lots if you decide to listen to some of the mindfulness CDs or apps), *it's just noticing what turns up, and not wanting to change anything in any way.*

Perhaps it's easier to tell you what mindfulness isn't

- Mindfulness is not watching a sunset and becoming stressed because you can't get your camera to work. If you are feeling stressed here, mindfulness helps you notice what you are experiencing and the effect it is having on your body, your thoughts and your mood; indeed how it could affect the rest of your evening.
- Mindfulness is not imagining how much more wonderful this experience would be if you were thinner, had the right shoes, were with a different partner, were with somebody else altogether.
- Mindfulness is not drifting off to past sunsets or past lovers.
- Mindfulness is not longing for something or running away from something, or analysing the past and following the tempters of 'if only'.
- Mindfulness is not running ahead to plan more sunsets or grasping onto the conditions of the sunset or planning future sunsets. Mindfulness is not about leaping into the fertile land of

'What if there are no more sunsets or something happens to me so that I cannot see the sunset?' while beating yourself up for not being who you think you should be.

- And just to cement things, mindfulness is not you snapping at your companion for interrupting your thoughts as you try to make this a perfect moment.

No, mindfulness is not any of these things.

Mindfulness means turning up for this sunset – and only this one

No matter what happened before and what might happen next, you turn up to the sunset and allow yourself to be bathed in the momentousness of light, colour and form, to feel the soft opening of your body and heart as the beauty penetrates your awareness. Even if there is stress, or a longing to be thinner, or a plan for future sunsets, or some kind of sadness, sitting here with you as the sun goes down, mindfulness allows you to be both your life and your sunset. In other words, with mindfulness, it's impossible to miss out on the beauty that's around us.

Practise standing up meditation

Earlier we did a really good sitting down meditation. Now, let's try standing up meditation. Another of the four dignities, standing is a wonderful way to practise your mindfulness.

So, take a stand – your stand on life – by rising from where you sit and truly standing on your spot, on your feet. Feel the contact with the floor, and bring awareness to your breath in this moment. Follow your breathing, and invite kind curiosity about how you feel in this moment. You might feel discomfort at some point, so direct your breath to the site of unease and soften it by breathing into it. You can have your hands by your sides or you can hold them out in front of you as a kind of offering.

You won't necessarily be able to stand for very long, so just notice how long you feel you can stand for, allowing yourself to sit down again when you need to. Perhaps you can hold out for slightly longer than feels comfortable – to get to the edge of what feels possible for you in this moment. This is, after all, your edge, your possibility. Keep focusing on your breathing, and if thoughts distract you – as they will – bring your attention gently and firmly back to the breath.

Stand for as long as feels right, or time yourself for ten minutes. When you sit down again, bring some kindness to yourself and congratulate yourself for this very simple act of standing up and sitting back down. It's no small feat, this work on your feet, when you think about it.

Mindfulness is about remembering you're the one living this precious life

As you begin to practise mindfulness with our little exercises, you might even begin to recognize how quickly the habits you have built to protect yourself are set to automatic pilot. Although these habits are no longer necessary, you still find yourself tensing your body or fixing your mind, which can lead you to destructive reactive patterns when you are with others. Or you might recognize how much energy you take up, and the astonishing array of things you will do, to avoid certain feelings when you are alone or still. Given how many years it takes us to develop these damaging habits, it is obvious it will take time and effort to undo or replace them with healthier living or coping systems.

We're seeing these habits as (at least potentially) the cause of stress; certainly, they're going to help us solve the crime. Mindfulness is the thing that will help us see through ourselves to the truth of our stress. And in that quiet place of mindfulness we can find rest, repair and resolve. Mindfulness, let's say, is fascinated by your habits, even if you aren't.

That brings us right back to the problem of a definition

I say problem, but we could also call it an opportunity. The opportunity to define mindfulness is helped by its original meaning. Mindfulness comes originally from the Pali word for 'awareness' and in this context belongs to the Buddhist tradition. A whole book could be spent talking about this and the brave innovators who have brought the major concepts of mindfulness to the West over the past two centuries. We might also acknowledge that many of the major concepts of mindfulness can be found in the contemplative traditions of all the world's religions: a concern with transforming the body and thoughts from a reactive ego to a more centred self, free of the propaganda of the mind and grasping. But we're getting ahead of ourselves. For now, let's just enjoy this thought: mindfulness is awareness.

Enter stage left the star of modern mindfulness, the inspirational Jon Kabat-Zinn

Probably the best-known pioneer of mindfulness is Jon Kabat-Zinn. Originally a biochemist and a meditator, in the 1980s he created what he called (and what is still called) the eight-week Mindfulness-Based Stress Reduction course. This book is very much inspired by this original eight-week course – Lorraine is a teacher of it, Philip has been a student of it, and we are both regular practitioners. If you've never done the eight-week course, we hope this book inspires you to give your nearest one a try. There are details at the end of how to find your nearest course, and they're available online or over the telephone too.

The eight-week course is a systematic course of eight two-hour meetings and a silent all-day retreat, alongside daily meditative homework

Jon Kabat-Zinn first presented the course for patients in his teaching hospital in Massachusetts who could no longer be helped. In other words, these were patients who had been told to go away and learn to live with pain or life-threatening disease that could not be cured. Kabat-Zinn devised the course to help his patients live around the edges of their pain – on that restless edge that flickers – and recognize the wholeness, centredness and connection within.

In just a short time, research on the course showed almost miraculous results. Kabat-Zinn became the talented catalyst who brought together cutting-edge science and neuroscience with the ancient wisdom drawn from many of the world's religions (primarily at that time Buddhism) in a beautiful and demonstrably effective union, which sent ripples of recognition throughout the whole world.

Kabat-Zinn's work recognized that many of us were struggling to cope with the ever-increasing demands of the modern world, using defence mechanisms unchanged since the time of cavepeople.

In the UK, the pioneers come from the world of psychology. Mark Williams, now at Oxford University, together with Zindel Segal and John Teasdale, whose background is in cognitive behavioural therapy, began researching the difficult territory of recurrent depression. Through work with Kabat-Zinn they devised the second main eight-week mindfulness course – called Mindfulness-Based Cognitive Therapy – which, research shows, has achieved excellent results in preventing relapse into depression. Since these two key eight-week courses were created, different expressions of mindfulness have sprouted all over the world and are all demonstrating that mindfulness practices work.

In this book, we take key elements of these fantastic eight-week courses, and offer them to you

Nevertheless, this book isn't a substitute for attending an eight-week course yourself. But perhaps even more important than reading the book or attending an eight-week course is for you to explore – in your own time and with great care – your own relationship with your body and your breath, and how you and they relate to your stress.

Finding your own path to mindfulness is part of the point. You can do it right here, right now.

But do take care. The great thing about doing this work with a trained professional is that he or she can help you with any difficulties that may arise. So when you read this book, just know that you can do as much or as little as you like; and ultimately look out for yourself during all this, asking yourself at any time, *What do I need? How can I support myself?* Put the book down if it's getting a bit too much or if you need to make a cup of mindful tea.

Practise lying down meditation

So we've had a go at sitting down meditation and standing up meditation; now let's try our hand at lying down meditation. Also known as the body scan, this is one of the most well-known mindfulness positions – the dignities – and is a core practice of the eight-week Mindfulness-Based Stress Reduction programme.

With this one, lie down in a safe spot that's comfortable – perhaps with a mat beneath you and a cushion under your head. Nothing in mindfulness need cause pain! Though pain is most welcome, of course, we try to minimize any extra pain when we set up our mindfulness experiments. Now that you are lying down, let your hands and feet flop gently apart and have your head facing up, perhaps supported by a pillow. Shut your eyes and begin to notice your breathing, not changing it, but simply noticing how you breathe in this moment.

Lying down meditation can last any amount of time, but a classic body scan – it is worth noting – takes about 45 minutes. In whatever time you have in this moment, start to bring awareness to the big toe of your left foot. You can even send – metaphorically of course – your breath to the big toe of your left foot by breathing down into it. Notice how it feels to be a big toe on the left foot. What is life like down here? What is the inside of the toe like? Can you feel it touching any other toes? This kind of enquiry is what you'll do now with every part of your entire body, because in the body scan we literally scan our whole body to check in with each part, and we assess, as a result, and mindfully, the whole of ourselves.

So we move from the big toe on the left foot to the little toe, to the toes in between, to the top and bottom of the left foot, to the ankle, to the shin, to the calf muscles, to the knee, to the thighs, to the crotch and genitals and buttocks, all the way down to the right foot and leg, up again to the small of the back, the upper back, the belly, the chest, the neck, the left and right arms and hands and fingers, then up to the head, mouth, nose, eyes, eyebrows – how does it feel to be an eyebrow today? – and up to the forehead, the brain, the top of the head and the hair. You might segue between part and whole; sometimes you'll be focusing on parts of the leg, sometimes you'll shine a light on the whole of the leg (which is also a part of the whole body).

Now focus on being an entire body, breathing and noticing and feeling and just letting it all go in this moment. The body scan is a wonderful practice, though it does take practice. We'll come back to it, but for now really enjoy lying down in this moment. Come back whenever you can, or feel free to chill out down there for a bit longer.

A little background on Lorraine's experience of mindfulness

I came to the eight-week Mindfulness-Based Stress Reduction course through the University of Bangor ten years ago and have been incorporating it into my work as a psychotherapist and teacher (I teach mindfulness) for the past eight years. I have been a therapist for almost 30 years and in this time have been trained in, and received therapy from, many different traditions. I have also been a long-term meditator for many years in the Buddhist tradition, with smatterings of Sufism and Hinduism. I gained an enormous amount from this practice but still would find myself falling into times when I had a searing feeling of dread and fear, and I had difficulty keeping my body steady in times of stress, even though I felt my mind was OK. Also, for most of my adult life, I have struggled with sleep. After my first eight-week mindfulness course I felt different, more in control of myself and my reactions to my life.

I learnt to turn with curiosity towards whatever sensation I was feeling in my body

I know it might sound so simple but I learnt not to assume how I felt. It *might not be* fear or dread. I was learning what we call **affect regulation**. Over time I discovered that the terrible feelings of dread I would experience seemingly out of nowhere most evenings were in fact my blood sugar level dropping about an hour after my regular habit of over-indulging in chocolate. The chocolate habit has not gone altogether, but I have managed to stop my mind interpreting the sensation as dread and running off in a million different neural circuits to remind me of every possible threat in life, leaving me desperate.

From the continual practice of tuning into my body and, in some instances, recognizing what is there (not what I think is there) I have been able to catch my body before it twists into the knot of stressfulness. And the same too goes for my thoughts: it is *I* who have control over *them*, not vice versa. I learnt the obvious fact that we cannot choose what thoughts ping into our brain, but we can choose what we do with them.

My mindfulness practice helped me spot my stress

I learnt I could turn towards those terrible patterns of shame I would plough into whenever I made a mistake. Instead of drowning in the chemicals of shame, I was learning – through mindfulness – to be compassionate, kind and curious to the automatic response of defensiveness, to the annihilating thoughts that I no longer deserved to exist. I learnt that this was the only way to take real responsibility and choose the response that would best allow me to go forward. I noticed my avoidance habits when I was turning against feelings or thoughts I did not want to feel, the thousands of pounds I had spent on trinkets and the hours of wasted time following the distraction of buying and worrying.

Most importantly for me I learnt how to turn up

With mindfulness – using these little practices we're showing you – I learnt how to turn up and really recognize beauty in the world around us. By truly tuning in, I was keeping my reward circuits switched on. I learnt that I can cultivate happiness; that – as Jane Fonda tells us – the only thing which is not on a trajectory of decay in this world is the human spirit.

Your mind will wander – don't worry

Throughout all these little mindful experiments we invite you do, you will likely find that your mind wanders while you're trying to focus on your breathing or on the inner sensation of a body part. This is going to happen; don't worry; there's nothing you can do to stop it. It's a good thing! You're alive, you're curious. Your mind wants to go exploring. So you simply invite the mind back to whatever it is you are focusing on in this moment – be it your breath or your contact with the earth. And you do this once, ten times or 80,000 times, no matter what. Each time you bring your attention back is another opportunity to explore how to live a full and possibility-rich life.

Mindfulness has taught me to be centred, kind and connected

It truly is a miracle. You learn that the world is the way you see it, not necessarily the way it is; that we have the power to change the negative spiral of false perception. With practice we realize that we have a choice about how we tune into the world and we can tune into that station so much more wisely and compassionately.

Philip has a similar story in terms of the benefits of mindfulness

I'm not a therapist or a mindfulness teacher (though one day I'd love to teach it), I'm a writer, and I sometimes run writing groups using bits I've learned from mindfulness. Mindfulness became crucial to me after I attended a friend's funeral and came to a huge and – for me personally – difficult realization. As I stood looking at the closed coffin of my gorgeous friend, I realized that her beautiful body was *in there*, and that my body was – in a similar way, but different obviously – *out here*. I remember looking at my body and at the coffin and wishing my friend could have her body back, my friend who had lived her life to the full through her beautiful embodiment. It felt as if I wasn't *here* as much as she wasn't *there*. It was as if, aged 31, I had only just realized I had a body.

I felt bad for ignoring my own body

That was in December. The following January I made a resolution to live the whole year in a full-bodied way. That meant embracing everything, every challenge, every tiny activity with the fullness of my body. Like a full-bodied wine, I wanted my body to be rich with experience. If I stubbed my toe, I zoomed into the feeling (as much as that is possible right after you stub your toe). I went wild swimming, I swung from a trapeze, I took up dance. I walked everywhere. I sat quietly in my room and just listened to what was happening to me. I tried to be a better brother, uncle, son, boyfriend.

I remember being amazed that the word *listen* is an anagram of *silent*

It didn't take me long to realize I was already on the path to practising mindfulness. I'm not bigging myself up by saying that. I hope I'm just emphasizing how naturally mindfulness came to me as a philosophy and a method. I was ready for it and it was ready for me. So I took to mindfulness – my mindfulness – like a duck to water. That doesn't mean I loved every moment of it, that I always looked forward to the group mindfulness sessions, that I didn't find the body scan boring at times, that I didn't fall asleep during sitting meditations, that I didn't occasionally burst into laughter during group meditation, or cry my eyes out while Lorraine led a sitting. Not at all. Mindfulness is – like almost anything in life, it seems – difficult. Difficult, but worth it. Mindfulness, in a way, is all about difficulty. So it has an inbuilt structure that enables you to cope with the difficulties it presents. Never give up, as my wise mum and dad have taught me.

Practise a three-minute dignity

Lots of the mindfulness books out there include an exercise like this, so it's not new, but we felt it was important for you to have a quick and easy way to bring mindfulness into your everyday life, inside and alongside the stresses and strains of modern living.

We call this a three-minute dignity. You've already read about the sitting, standing and lying down meditations, three of the different positions also known as dignities. We love this idea of dignity so much that we reckon it's possible to bring in a bit of dignity to any part of your busy life. Here's how it goes. Do this in whatever position, or dignity, you like.

Stop Simply bring yourself to your centre in this moment. Whatever you are doing, stop and allow yourself to notice your breathing. If you can't literally stop (sometimes the external things that are causing you stress mean you can't), metaphorically stop by centring yourself and finding your inner stillness in the speed and rush of events. Stop and breathe. Do this for a minute.

Look Next, look around you and notice what you see. Bring kind eyes to the objects of your attention. Now do the same but this time bring your looking inside yourself. Notice how you are making contact with the floor. Notice how your body feels – its proprioception (where each part is in space) and its interoception (the feeling of insideness). Send some special breathing down to any painful or intense sensations. Look outwards and look inwards for another minute.

Listen For the final minute, listen to any sounds in this moment. They could be the sounds of cars or other people's voices, whether pulling you away from this moment or not. Just notice them for what they are and don't try to follow them. Then bring your listening inwards. Listen to the thoughts inside your head. Hear what they have to say. Observe them and try not to follow them. Just let them be, as thoughts, not pied pipers about to whisk you away. Listen outwards, and listen inwards, for this final minute. And after this third minute, allow yourself to come gently back to yourself as a whole creature with a full and fabulous life ahead of you.

There. You've done a three-minute dignity and you can now bring it to any part of your day. To bring dignity to your stress, and indeed your life, in this way is beautiful.

Back to that last point: mindfulness is about difficulty because any difficulty can be approached with mindfulness

- Scared of a meeting tomorrow? Bring mindfulness to it. Sit with your thoughts about tomorrow in the present moment. That's the only time you've got.
- Frustrated with a friend who is ignoring something important? Brilliant. Breathe into it and bring mindfulness to it. How might you *respond* to your friend now (instead of *reacting* to him or her)?
- Overworked and underpaid? In your next mindfulness session, ask each part of your body how it's feeling; is it feeling the same? Might there be other words to describe yourself? What positive action might you be able to take now? What is your Job with a capital J (as Jon Kabat-Zinn says), the one that the universe is calling for you to step up to?

- Are you exhausted? Rest. Bring kind and generous curiosity to your tiredness. Perhaps you just need to sleep – so sleep. Perhaps you can make enquiries, in which case meditate a little while and ask your body about its tiredness before you run a soothing bath and go to bed.

And joy too – mindfulness of joy is just as important

Mindfulness is often discussed in relation to stress and depression and things that cause us pain, but that's only half the story. We need to become mindful throughout our experience:

- Excited about a new job? Sit in stillness and let the excitement settle. Feel the excitement pour into all areas of your body. Is it truly excitement? Are there any other words to describe it? If it is truly excitement, be truly excited. If it's something else, allow yourself to make your experience more complex and subtle. You need to slow down to be that various, but it's possible and rewarding.
- Are you over the moon about meeting up with your friends? Lovely. Mindfulness can help as you approach the meeting to keep you clear headed, practise your kindness skills and cope with the passing of time; after all, this lovely moment, too, will pass.
- Are you, in this moment, unbelievably happy? You don't need to meditate to be mindful. Just be unbelievably happy in this moment. Enjoy it. Being the very thing you are being is exactly the point about mindfulness – whether you experience joy or pain, stress or calm.

In a nutshell, the skills and insights you learn from mindfulness can help you focus and be more productive, and can lead you to a deep centred place with a sense of connection to yourself, others and the world around you. In a secular world mindfulness can connect you to your place in the order of things as a member of the silent revolution making ourselves, and the world, a better, calmer, safer, happier, more appreciative place for all. And if you are religious, it connects up with the heart of all religions' enquiry into contemplation and connectivity, whether you're a Christian or a Hindu, a Jew, a Muslim, a Pagan or even a Jedi (Yoda knew a thing or two about mindfulness).

Mindfulness recognizes that the most positive change is not made by criticism and punishment but by warm, friendly, kind curiosity

When we discover all the tricks of distraction and resistance the mind plonks in our way, we are learning to respond to it with firmness, bringing the mind back when it wanders off with a kinder, softer inner voice that is on our side rather than against us. Stress-resilient people have a supportive inner voice, not a critical voice that wants to punish them. Their inner voice is clear and responsible but compassionate towards themselves. Cultivating this voice is at the heart of mindfulness.

With mindfulness, we notice the minutiae of our movements

We notice how often the mind will limit us or push us to things the body may not agree with. We learn to be responsive to the needs of our body and gently encourage it. Flexibility in goals is a vital part of the resilient character. Slowly we are learning that if we become fixed and rigid in our thinking we will always be living in the doom-laden area of deficit: being too fat, not having the right job, etc. Here we are entering the territory of *if only*, which does not get us where we want to be any quicker. In fact it fills us with stress and demotivates us from believing we can go where we need to go at all.

Practise mindful walking

The fourth dignity is mindful walking. Unlike other kinds of walking, it isn't the aim of mindful walking to get anywhere. In this exercise, you will simply walk slowly – very slowly – back and forth, while you attend to yourself with awareness and great generosity of spirit. So throw yourself some rope while you're doing this funny act of walking: trust, trust, trust.

> You don't need much space, and it's advisable to be somewhere private, where you won't be interrupted. All you need is a bit of space in which you can walk backwards and forwards, probably something like 10 steps in each direction but perhaps even fewer. Quantity doesn't matter so much as the quality of your experience of each step. With mindful walking you simply slow walking down to its basic components.
>
> Lift one foot and slowly let it move in its arc, while the other foot waits. Really feel how that foot feels in the moment of the arc towards the next patch of earth. As it touches ground, lift the other foot, and again zoom in on the feelings of lifting, lifting, lifting and then placing down, placing down, placing down. Repeat this until you have walked about 10 steps. Then turn around, stand with dignity for a moment, and return the way you came. All the while, notice your breathing and how your breathing and walking go hand in hand. You can even slow your breathing down so that you breathe and move one step forward at the same pace.
>
> Once you have walked back and forth a few times like this, experiment by changing the pace of your walking, changing how you hold your hands and arms and how you breathe. Why not try walking and saying *Thank* when the left foot touches the ground and *You* when the right foot touches the ground – *Thank . . . You . . . Thank . . . You . . .* – so that you walk in gratitude?
>
> When you come to a final stop, shut your eyes, breathe into your new standing position and do a few minutes of standing meditation to finish off the session.

As with the other dignities, you can do this as a three-minute dignity during your day or whenever you approach your stress.

With mindfulness practice, we can simply be

We recognize how we can sit still (or stand still or walk slowly) and notice awareness as it arises in the breath. We notice the body's sounds, and we begin to get a hold on thoughts and see them as mental activity rather than as the whole of us. The words or thoughts that come up are no more your mind than clouds are the clear blue sky, as Jon Kabat-Zinn says.

This is the art of watching our thoughts like weather

Here we begin to untie the knot of automatic pilot thoughts. We learn to recognize the difference between an event and our interpretation of that event and how our thoughts and actions radiate from the interpretation, not the facts.

Let's go *Whoa there*, and look at that again:

- There is a difference between the event itself and our interpretation of the event.
- Our thoughts and actions radiate from the interpretation of the event, not the facts.

If we do this good work of separating event from interpretation, we learn how our interpretations can be affected by our moods and how our moods can be affected by our interpretations. We see too how our moods are caught up in our thoughts, sensations and emotions and are followed by an automatic pilot impulse to act.

Resilient people – people who might have a mindfulness practice – pause before they jump to conclusions, because there's an awful lot going on, right?

One of the forefathers of British mindfulness, Alan Watts, turned this idea into a beautiful, funny poem

There was a young man who said 'Though
It seems that I know that I know,

What I would like to see,
Is the I that knows Me
When I know that I know that I know.'

With mindfulness, we learn how important it is to keep our eyes and ears open to the world around us

We learn how to respond to pleasurable events – even the smallest things like the feel of the sun on our face or the beauty of a daffodil. We notice that, in our act of noticing, our body responds by gently opening a little, giving us a small boost of chemicals to help us feel good and resilient. We feel calm and our thoughts for a while might even be still; we notice too how we can recapture this feeling simply by bringing it to mind.

Keep a mindful journal

One way of integrating all this mindfulness stuff into your life is by keeping a mindful journal. This is particularly useful if you experience stress. You can use your mindful journal to write down any stresses you are experiencing in the moment, or in the day, or in the past week. Writing them down makes them more real. We can work with them. To paraphrase the judo maestro and pioneer of bodywork, Moshe Feldenkrais, we can only change what we're doing when we know what we're doing. Writing itself can also be a mindfulness meditation and can help you expand your capacity for self-awareness, compassion and resilience. Philip has written more on this in the Sheldon Mindfulness book, *Keeping a Journal*, which is full of tips on how to bring mindful journal practice into your everyday life.

If you're curious about the world, it's difficult to be anxious

When you learn mindfulness, you learn how thoughts can become a rapid stream of negativity and catastrophe and rigidity, all because of the way we interpret them. When you learn mindfulness you are learning choice and the responsibility you have to take in order to recognize choice.

We learn that the world exists purely in the way we interpret it, and that how we interpret it will affect our mood and productivity. Our muscle of awareness is now strong enough that we are able to choose to keep focus and not be swept away by thoughts or feelings. We have learnt the great secret of resilient people – that you can cultivate courage, happiness and resilience by simply tuning into the right station and out of the wrong wavelengths.

Stress-resilient people are not afraid of strong feelings or difficult thoughts

With mindfulness we are able to face the difficult things without being consumed by them. It is said that most addictions begin with a need to run away from a big feeling, maybe one that we first ran away from when we were a small baby. Before our brain even had the capacity to give it a cognitive meaning, or our hippocampus the ability to turn it into a memory, at some time a thought or an emotion settled in us and we felt we had to avoid it or it would destroy us or the world as we knew it. So, over time, we adapt our behaviour in some wonderfully creative ways to help us avoid such feelings and thoughts; some of these adaptations serve us well, but many (possibly most) really don't. The constant state of hyper-alertness we develop in order to continually fend off the thoughts is exhausting and can get in our way, stopping us from becoming all that we have the potential to be.

With mindfulness, we are given an opportunity to go towards stress

We do this not by following tangled thoughts but by recognizing our lived experience in the body. We have the courage to go towards these feelings, and get below them; we realize that feelings are actually a cluster of physical sensations and thoughts that will grow and grow if we feed them and gather in strength if we continue to push them away. The odd thing is that most of these fears are no longer valid, even if they ever were; they were products of a child's mind without the full story to make sense of them. They often boil down to feeling unworthy, unloveable, angry or sad. Some have the potential to drop us into a pit of shame.

Having learnt how to regulate some of these difficult feelings by breathing gently and turning towards ourselves with kindness and acceptance, we are learning that our demons are not so scary, and are usually not telling us the truth. Even if we did make errors, or behaved in a way we now feel shameful about, we can never make amends by hating ourselves and running away.

Instead, mindfulness teaches us to look our demons in the eye without being destroyed, and watch them dissipate. We gain the courage to own up to things and make a choice to live our lives to the fullest, with much more responsibility and connection. We can learn how to identify our avoidance or coping mechanisms and choose the useful rather than the destructive ones in the future.

Mindfulness builds resilience in you

And resilience gives you purpose and meaning. We begin to feel ourselves as more centred and learn to willingly swap to the being rather than the doing mode whenever we feel a destructive, reactive pattern setting in. With mindfulness, we are like the mountain, able to notice the weather conditions changing around us, the night turning to day; mindfulness gives us something solid to hold onto rather than being jostled by every thought, feeling or event that slips into our awareness.

With mindfulness we learn to recognize some of our automatic pilot thoughts . . .

. . . and how they connect to a million others that lead us down very difficult ruminative pathways that will not be helped (in fact they will only be worsened) by the rumination. This, of course, is not to say that we don't need thoughts, or patterns of thoughts, that help us make sense of the world and our lives. It just means, from a mindfulness point of view, that we need to be discerning as to which thoughts we listen to and follow them only when the time is right. With this practice, we can also cultivate the soft, gentle, non-judgemental voice within. This helps us realize that the world has the meaning we give it.

Viktor Frankl, in his book *Man's Search for Meaning*, which chronicled his time in a concentration camp during the Second World War, illustrates this beautifully. He realized that in order to survive he had to find meaning in what was happening to him and could not surrender by allowing himself to see himself through his captors' eyes. He could also see that having a sense of meaning would often make the difference between whether prisoners survived or not. He came out with these wonderful sayings:

If you know why,
you can put up with any how

and

Man's last freedom is the freedom
to choose our attitude.

I think we can see that this is the same for us. If we see the work we do as drudgery, and constantly resent what our job requires of us, our mood will be constantly low. If, however, we can see our job as an opportunity to help us connect, and can take the time on the commute into work to enjoy reading our book, or looking at the scenery, or listening to those very noisy kids, then our sense of self and enjoyment in the world will flourish.

When we learn mindfulness, we learn how to incorporate breathing spaces throughout our days and discover how to help ourselves when we feel overwhelmed or on the cusp of a plunge into negativity. And most of all we learn more and more to cultivate our inner best friend, who does not let us off the hook but has a deep belief in our good intentions and huge worth. With mindfulness, we tune into the things that nourish us.

It's not stress, we'll discover in the next chapter, that will kill us, but our response to it

This is ground-breaking stuff, it really is. We can start to plan how we take this learning into our lives, for the rest of our lives. We realize how much beauty there is in the world, if only we can bring our dignity to it.

3

What stress is and why it's one of the most interesting things about you

You already know what stress is

In a funny way, it's one of the only words in the English language that doesn't need defining. We just know, don't we, when we are stressed – or 'stressed out', as we might also say. Stress is:

- having too much work to do in too little time;
- failing at something you really want to achieve;
- being confronted by something, or someone, you're scared of;
- being unable to change something you desperately want to change;
- living with a long-term debilitating condition;
- carrying too many bags of shopping home by yourself and then having to cook a meal for you and your three children, before writing a job application once you've put the kids to bed.

You get the idea.

Do a three-minute dignity

We're about to talk about stress. This could get stressful. So let's practise the three-minute dignity we learned earlier.

> As we are about to consider stress – and you specifically are about to consider your own relationship with your stress – try to simply let your mind and body be. Stop what you're doing and find your centre. Breathe in and out, noticing the gap in between your in- and out-breaths. Look around you and within you. Notice your contact with the earth. Listen for sounds and, inside you, have kind ears that hear your thoughts but do not follow them. Just let yourself be in this moment.
>
> Now, in this moment, allow the words *My Stress* to filter into your consciousness. Hold them inside your body, or outside your body, and see how the words affect you. Notice any changes in your body. Breathe into any areas of intensity as you hold the words *My Stress* inside or outside your body. Now let the words go. Detach from them and sit in the simplicity of the present moment.

The classic idea of stress: it is bad for you

According to the classic idea, stress is my experience of a bad thing and its effects on my body (which are also bad). So stress is bad, the story goes.

Mindfulness has another version of stress that it wants to tell you. Mindfulness says that, actually, stress is another opportunity with which to explore life and live fully and wholly. Stress is something I can take to the mindfulness workroom, as it were. It is something I can examine with care and kindness. In a way, my stress is the very thing that makes me *Me*. It is possibly the most interesting thing about me. How I respond mindfully to my stress – rather than how I react – is the thing. It is practice for living life fully. Stress is life. Why would we want to get rid of stress, even if we could? To get rid of stress would be to get rid of life.

Wait for it: stress can be good

Or perhaps more accurately: stress is neither good nor bad. What is good or bad is how we respond to stress. And how we respond to stress really is the thing here. Imagine a man coming home with the shopping. Here are two ways of looking at his situation from his point of view. Compare this way . . .

'Ugh, I hate carrying all these shopping bags. I'm so tired after my day at work. Why do I deserve this? And there we go, one of my bags has just broken. Great! I'm not surprised, this always happens to me. And when I get back, ugh, I've got to cook food for that lot. And then I have to put them to bed – will they ever stop jumping up and down on their beds? – and write another bloody application for a job I probably won't get anyway. I don't know why I bother.'

with this way:

'As I walk home along this beautiful river, I notice my body aches in reaction to the bags I'm carrying. Fair enough. I'm going to take a moment to rest, notice my breathing, and really feel what I'm feeling. One of my bags has just broken but I'm going to just be with that and in a moment try and make do. And here I find myself chuckling, because I can't seem to pick up all the bags now. There we go. When I get back I'll get the kids to help with putting some of this stuff away and then we'll make a really simple dinner together. They'll be so excited to see me and I'm lucky I get to spend time with them. After stories at bedtime (and perhaps I'll allow a couple of bounces up and down on the beds beforehand), I'll try and write a job application. It might be possible or it might not. I won't beat myself up about it.'

OK, these are both caricatures of inner monologues, but the point is made: it is possible to see the same situation in more than one way. When we bring mindfulness to our stress, we can open up some space for ourselves, for joy (like seeing the river) and for kindness to ourselves ('I won't beat myself up about it').

With mindfulness of stress, we shift from 'got to' to 'get to'

One of the main shifts of mindset between the two monologues is this: we go from 'I've *got* to do this thing' to 'I *get* to do this thing'. Think of all the times you've stressed out about something and described it in terms of *got* rather than *get*:

- I've got to do the washing up.
- I've got to make a speech in front of 100 strangers.
- I've got to go on an aeroplane.

'Got' is the past of 'get', so with this shift we literally bring ourselves into the present. See how, with mindfulness, we can take a fresh look at these three stressful activities:

- I get to do the washing up – and explore how the soap suds feel against my skin and use the moment of standing up to notice how I'm breathing.
- I get to make a speech in front of 100 strangers, and explore how that feels, me standing in front of so many eyes; I'll zoom into the feelings in my legs and I'll take some deep breaths to help me slow down my speaking and really look at people as I talk to them.
- I get to go on an aeroplane and explore how I feel; I know I'm scared of flying but I have to fly for my job so I may as well confront it now. I've done some training for this so I feel prepared, and now I get to practise my new skills.

Write down three things that you recently found stressful

List them in whatever order you like. They can vary in magnitude from the tiniest moment of stress to the biggest traumatic ongoing period of your life. Make sure you're comfortable doing this, of course, we don't want to add to your stress. Write down what made you feel stressed but don't worry about writing too much. Just point to it, as it were, with words. Now look back at your list. Is there any way of shifting from the idea of 'I've got to do something' to 'I get to do something'? Is there any way you could look afresh at your stress?

Be careful here. We don't want you to ignore your stress or redefine it out of existence. It's still stress. We're just trying to find the full-ness in the stressfulness. We want you to take a closer look. Is it really all bad? Can we find some good in it too? You can write about your stress at any time. Journalling is a fantastic way of working with stress and has been shown by scientists like James Pennebaker to be conducive to physical health and mental well-being.

Rather than stress, there are stress factors and stress responses

There's actually no such thing as 'stress'. This is worth teasing out a bit. Though it's important not to deny the existence of stress – it's very real – what we talk about when we talk about stress is in fact two different things: **stress factors** and **stress responses**. The word stress, in a way, is shorthand for 'All the things to do with stress factors and stress responses'.

Stress factors are things 'out there', like jobs, public speaking, not having enough money, ill health. Stress responses are things 'in here': panicking, running away, feeling hot, and so on. Your stress response is how you respond to the stress factor in any given moment.

So with mindfulness of stress, we redefine stress, and our relationship to stress

There are plenty of definitions of stress, though they all go back to Dr Hans Selye, whose work using rats in the 1950s is instrumental in our current understanding of stress in humans.

Selye defined stress as 'the nonspecific response of the organism to any pressure or demand'. That's quite a broad remit for stress!

You experience pressure right now – the pressure of this book against your hands: feeling stressed? But it's a good definition actually: like stress, it is broad and general, and it emphasizes the fact that stress is a natural part of life and cannot be avoided. It does however also suggest that everything might be stress – that life itself is stress! This is possible, but in order for the stress to be really meaningful when we do experience it, we have to allow ourselves the chance that we're not actually experiencing stress in all given moments.

Another stress researcher, Dr Richard Lazarus, argues that stress is more a transaction between a person and his or her environment. Lazarus defines stress as 'a particular relationship between the person and the environment that is appraised by the person as taxing or exceeding his or her resources and endangering his or her well-being'.

This transactional idea of stress is useful inasmuch as we can use techniques like mindfulness as one of the resources Lazarus mentions here. In other words, stress is something we can get better at doing. I like this definition of stress, though it still leaves me on the lookout.

For the purposes of this book, we really like the definition of stress put forward by Kelly McGonigal in her book, *The Upside of Stress*:

Stress is what arises when something you care about is at stake.

Looked at in this way, stress becomes much more a human experience – rather than, say, a 'nonspecific response' or a 'transaction'. To talk about stress in terms of what we care about is to radically reappraise our understanding of stress, and it's that understanding of stress – based on what we care about – that we want to argue for in this book. Mindfulness is very interested in what you care about, so it's interested in your stress. Your stress – what you care about – is one of the most interesting things about you. Keep being yourself, in other words, and honour yourself by building stress-resilience in whatever way works for you.

What each of us considers stressful, and the way in which we respond to stressful situations, is different for everybody – and of course every body

We can be stressed both by things that are unpleasant and things that are pleasant. We become stressed when our system feels overwhelmed by an upcoming event, which can be either pleasant or unpleasant. Stress could be a butterfly flying too close to my hair (Lorraine says that if it's a bird doing the same, she'll go into cardiac arrest). Another person might find this a highly joyful or calming experience. So we are left with the fact that many of the things we find stressful physically, mentally, emotionally or even spiritually, are very subjective.

Stress is real but subjective

So what triggers the stress response in us is an internal stress factor (like worry) or an external stress factor (like workload) which we feel is about to overwhelm our system. If our system feels it cannot tolerate the event, our stress response will be triggered, causing a variety of symptoms.

What's really interesting is that our response to stress is more important than the thing that's stressing us

In other words, we can take control, because we can practise responding better; at least we can practise techniques like mindfulness, which help us review our stress-related mindset.

Studies show that how you view your stress is a function of the way you approach it and that you can actually change how you view your stress. In one such study, a group of women doing housework actually experienced benefits similar to those of exercise if – compared to women who didn't have that opinion – they initially *thought* that housework was as beneficial as exercise. In other words, how you interpret the facts is important; how you see something could be how it will turn out. The implications for us in practising mindfulness of stress are huge: will we see a particular activity as stressful or we will see it as being beneficial (giving us new skills, helping us be courageous and so on)? None of this is to deny stress factors, but it is to suggest that no matter who you are, you can work on your stress response – and mindfulness as a technique can help you do that.

Of course, our stress response system goes back to us being cavepeople

Our stress response system was originally designed for our cavemen and women ancestors who needed a keen response mechanism when dealing with predators. It simply hasn't been updated to deal with twenty-first century stressors.

In the classic account of stress (say in response to an attack by a sabre-toothed tiger), you can do one of three things:

1 Flight: you can run like hell.
2 Fight: you can throw spears and take a chance of warding off and protecting your dependants.
3 Freeze: you play dead and freeze all your perceptions to lighten the trauma of being eaten. At the most extreme, with terrifying situations where there is no chance of escape, you might just make yourself numb to the situation altogether by becoming completely absent (called dissociating) and go into another time or place in your head in the hope that you will survive.

When the danger is physical, the stress response is all well and good. If you survive, you survive.

What's happening in your body during all this stress?

We won't go into too much detail, but suffice to say, when the body perceives a threat the limbic system (the part of the brain that retains emotional memory and activates emotional response) sends a signal to the hypothalamus to start up the stress response, depositing a rush of chemicals in its wake. To most of us this will mean physical reactions to the stress usefully made to put the body and mind into a state of hyper-alertness in order to prepare to fight, take flight or freeze. You will recognize the symptoms:

- rapid heartbeat
- tense muscles
- focused thoughts on threat
- strong emotions
- the release of adrenalin creating a sense of dread, that butterfly sinking feeling.

Or you feel unable to think or react at all, literally rendering you powerless.

As soon as the threat is over (the sabre-toothed tiger has moved on), physical exhaustion will bring into action the body's parasympathetic nervous system, after which things calm down and the disregulated state returns to equilibrium. This is classically understood stress and it affects all of us.

List your body's responses to recent stressful experiences

At the top of one column on a piece of paper, write down the title, 'The facts'. Above the next column, write down the title, 'The body'. In a third column, write down the title, 'The emotions'. Now either use the three stressful moments we mentioned earlier, or come up with some new ones, and write down the *facts* of each (what happened from an objective point of view), how it affected your *body*, and how you experienced it subjectively through the *emotions*. This will help you to separate the stress factor from the stress response and spot any continuities or divergences in your bodily and emotional responses. It will also help you observe your overall relationship with stress. Can you see anything interesting going on?

But it's not all sabre-toothed tigers

In fact, most stress isn't, is it? Most of the time – well, if we're lucky perhaps – we aren't under threat of meeting our maker. I can imagine that sort of situation is stressful, but most stress is much more nebulous. Most of the time in our world we perceive threat from internal senses of shame or fear of losing our sense of self or status, of being excluded on Facebook, and so on, and these threats do not have a resolution or off switch to allow the body to recover again.

As there are lots of types of stress factors, there are lots of types of stress responses

Let's have a look at them (these are again from Kelly McGonigal's brilliant book, *The Upside of Stress*):

The fight, flight and freeze response We've already looked at this. It's the classic story of stress, the one the cavepeople developed for us all those millennia ago. It's a useful way of thinking about stress, but how often are our lives in such danger? Of course, many people lead dangerous lives, but generally – in the modern world – our survival isn't on the line as it once was.

The excite and delight response Some stress is exhilarating and we go towards it. This is the kind of stress you might experience if you like jumping out of planes. You do it 'for the rush'. It's stress, but the kind of stress you willingly pay money to experience on a weekend.

The challenge response Lots of stress falls under this category. Our survival isn't on the line but we have to perform under pressure. This is the kind of stress you might experience at work, for example. You get some good chemical reactions when you do well, you feel focused but not fearful. You're up for it. Often associated with a craft or a skill, this is the kind of stress response you get when you're in the flow of things. You gain increased confidence, enhanced concentration and might even access your peak performance – though it can be stressful if you feel you're failing the challenge in some way.

The tend-and-befriend response If the fight-or-flight response is about you surviving, this response is about you trying to protect your community and the people around you. This kind of stress encourages you, you seek other people's support, you want to talk things over. Your stress response is to protect your tribe, share your feelings, talk and be listened to. You become a generator of courage in yourself and in other people. You want to defend your team.

The upshot of all this is fascinating, when you think about it. If we slow down enough, using our mindfulness practice, we can turn up to our stress and, instead of impulsively reacting, make a mindful decision how to proceed. We get to decide: now that I recognize the stress factor, which part of my stress response do I need the most?

- Do I fight?
- Do I run away?
- Do I freeze?
- Do I run up to it and shout *Yes!*?
- Do I engage more contemplatively?
- Do I connect with others around me?
- Do I find meaning in this situation?
- Do I grow as a person?

Stress can help you survive, but it can also help you challenge yourself, connect with others and grow

That's the key point here. Research shows that stress has a lot going, and growing, for it. It's why we reckon stress is one of the most interesting things about you. Stress isn't a one-way thing, it's always about you and your relationship to stress. It's funny, perhaps, to think about having a relationship to stress in the same way we have a relationship to our parents, brothers and sisters and friends. But we do have a relationship to stress, and that's the crux of the matter when it comes to mindfulness.

Do a three-minute dignity – and remember a time when stress felt good

Practise our simple meditation exercise: stop what you're doing and notice your breathing, look around you and inside yourself, listen to sounds and notice any thoughts (but don't follow them).

Then, once you have done this and cleared a space, remember a time when you were stressed, but it felt good. You might have been working on a team project, or trying for a baby, or walking up a mountain. Whatever you did, you experienced stress but you also overcame an obstacle and got through to the other side. You carried yourself forward. How did the victory feel? Was the stress useful at some level? Would you have felt how you did when you completed the challenge if you hadn't had the stress?

Why not do this exercise with a friend, too? It helps to share experiences like this. And if there isn't a friend at hand, and no one to telephone, why not write a letter to someone, telling them you're investigating your own relationship to stress and would they be interested to join in?

All we're saying is that mindfulness is a really useful tool for examining your relationship with stress

In those slowed-down moments, when you're following your breath, feeling your contact with the floor, noticing what you can hear and see, observing your thoughts as thoughts, you give yourself space to examine crucial things like your stress response. Your mindfulness practice helps you step outside yourself a wee while, helps you take a look at yourself, as if you are a detached, but kind, observer. With mindfulness – and no one says it's easy – you can hold your regular stress response in your arms and let yourself see it for what it is. In the stress-full moment, your mindfulness can help you slow down so that you become more spacious and respond, rather than react, to the stress factor. With mindfulness you 'get to do' things rather than feel you have 'got to do' them.

Some people seem more prone than others to negative stress responses

Why is that? It could be our genes; it could be the blueprint we developed as children. Our brain is pretty undeveloped when we arrive in the world. The basic mechanism is there but it is waiting to be formed in response to the environment in which we are born. If we are lucky and are given the privilege of a safe, secure society and emotionally stable carers, we have all the foundations for building a secure stress response. We will have been taught that when we cry, when we are hungry, lonely or sad, grown-ups will come to our aid and soothe and regulate us back to well-being, back to bodily regulation. In time this repeated assurance will help us to learn to self-regulate our system so that we can turn to other humans when we feel insecure or afraid.

How we respond to stress could go back to our early attachments

When we were little, if we were lucky, we made a secure enough attachment to basically trust in the human race and believe that we were loveable and worthy enough, just as we were, to be a valued and protected member of it. We will have been modelled healthy coping mechanisms for when the world gets a bit rocky and we will know how to behave in order to be accepted by the community in which we live, with enough confidence to be true to ourselves.

We will have been given a meaning system that helps us understand our place in the universe, and an empathy system to help us communicate our needs and pick up the needs of others. If we are really lucky we will have been given a core of beliefs that, no matter what we do or achieve, gives us a deep sense of self-trust and confidence that we have the potential to be whole, compassionate and loved enough. We will have the means to connect to each other and feel the stirrings of recognition and awe in poetry, art, music, a mountain or dance; feel connected to the world and the wonder of the universe.

When thoughts start to tear away at us we will have the means to bring ourselves back to a firm centre and reframe ourselves in the most useful way. We will trust that although we see terrible events on the news, we belong to an evolving world in which things can be done better; we can find our home in an active part of the silent revolution where personal ego makes place for a higher good and do what the rest of the creatures in our world do – live their lives to make their habitat and families as strong and secure as possible, without destroying the delicate ecosystem of our planet.

As you will probably see, most of us are not so lucky

And even if we are, the demands of the world we live in may well have interfered with the wiring so that we will have developed some rather distorted reactions. What's more, many of us may have some, but not all, or hardly any, or none at all of the above, so we learn to make creative adaptations in order to help us survive. It might be because of environmental, social or attachment issues that we have learnt not to trust others, the world or ourselves. All kinds of abuse, neglect, trauma and day-to-day conflicts can ebb away at our secure base and leave us not responding to the world the way it actually is but the way we think it is or fear it is. This can mean that our sense of threat or stress is activated at the slightest thing and we are constantly being flooded by hypervigilance and stress chemicals.

Practise mountain meditation

We've adapted this meditation from Jon Kabat-Zinn's work and it's truly wonderful to listen to him guide you through it on his famous mindfulness CDs, which are also available online. Mindfulness loves metaphors and I reckon one of the best ones is the invitation to sit – or indeed stand – like a mountain.

First, sit down with kindness and mindfulness, bringing awareness to your breathing. Notice your contact with the floor, any sounds around the room, the air touching your skin. Now that you have centred yourself, bring into your mind's eye a mountain you know – either through climbing it once, or through books, or from seeing it on television. Or of course you can make it up.

Now visualize this mountain, its strong foundations, its majestic height, its firmness and resilience. Imagine it in different seasons, with snow on its peak, with lush grass and trees round its base, with storms raging one minute, bright sun shining the next. Imagine the birds and the goats and cows with bells and the people who use this mountain on a daily basis. In amongst all the changes of life, the mountain has a firm and stable base, a presence, that persists, that is bigger and stronger than anything that can happen to it.

Holding this mountain in your mind's eye, you now bring the mountain inside, imagining you are mountain-like. You sit like a mountain. And like a mountain, nothing can spoil you. Things can happen on your surface, avalanches can occur, but you – the mountain – are left unscathed. You persist, you remain, you are resilient. As you sit and breathe like a mountain, see how this rests with you. Perhaps you even have a half-smile. Perhaps you enjoy this feeling? Or perhaps it feels like too much responsibility? Either way, just notice how it feels – ticking the thought, not following it.

And then, when you are ready, come out of your mountain pose, and find yourself in your normal sitting position, noticing how spacious you might be feeling and the quality of your breathing in this moment. Take your time before standing up and continuing your day. Look for opportunities to bring your mountain-like resilience into your day.

But there's good news: the brain is now seen as 'plastic'; we can all change, we can all work on our stress response

Neuroscience has given us the knowledge to explain why our systems become bundles of stress, which is translated into all types of anxiety and depression. However, another wondrous thing that it has taught us is that for the most part the brain is plastic and can be rewired. We know how the brain needs to be rewired to help us cope.

And this is why we are here today, writing this book: because when we put together everything that helps us be resilient to stress and life's ups and downs, when we look through the catalogue of our experiences and available antidotes, the best and most consistent is mindfulness.

Here's why mindfulness is so useful for stress

Mindfulness – as you can already tell – is about turning up to the present moment, which is the only moment stress really exists in. Even stress borne from memory of a stressful time is still stress experienced in the present moment. Mindfulness can do all sorts of things when it comes to stress, including:

- *Affect regulation*: mindfulness helps you pause the flood and bring the body back to a place of equilibrium.
- *Understanding the power of the body*: mindfulness enables you to recognize that the world is not the way it is but the way we perceive it to be. Here, mindfulness unties the knots of our automatic pilot reactions.
- *Flexibility of thinking and goals*: mindfulness gives you skills that enable you to be quick on your feet, because with mindfulness you aren't stuck on anything, you're up for anything.
- *Keeping reward centres open*: mindfulness helps you welcome all things, including rewards like pleasure.
- *Not avoiding but facing fears*: mindfulness is about going up close to difficulty, not running away from it. Even if our stress response is

to run away, we run away mindfully, we face our fears, we explore them (perhaps next time we won't run away, who knows?) as we run. With mindfulness, we don't hide anything.

- *Recognizing our destructive habits*: the way we think affects our immune system, sense of choice and autonomy: our mindfulness helps show us that how we perceive the world is how the world can be.

- *Sense of community and connection to the world, creative expression, spirit*: mindfulness helps you connect to a wider fabric and continuity, helping you to extend outwards in a more generous, grateful way.

Take a moment to let all this settle in before turning the page. Use this moment of transition between chapters to notice your breathing, your body's orientation towards the book and the world beyond it, the softness of your gaze. We'll look at lots more of this stuff in the next chapter, but for now explore as you find yourself in this moment. Ask yourself what you need, if you need anything at all; make a cup of mindful tea; take time to refresh and renew after all we've experienced in this chapter.

4

From stressfulness to mindfulness – going deeper

Mindfulness is yours for the taking

Mindfulness is both a technique involving skills that can be learned and practised and an entire way of life. In this book you are getting an inkling of what those practices are – the dignities of sitting, standing, lying down and walking – and you might be reflecting on how to bring them into your everyday life.

It might be possible to live mindfully all the time, but let's not get too stressed about that. If we can't do it in this moment, we can't do it in this moment. Isn't noticing you're not being mindful a kind of being mindful, anyway?

Let's practise mindfulness so that we are aware of it and it can guide us as much as is humanly possible. The emphasis here is on the word *human*.

The answer to the question about how to bring mindfulness to your stress is simple

It's both terribly simple and terribly difficult (sorry). To bring mindfulness to your stress, you just need to build your mindfulness practice. The key thing is to practise, practise, practise. That means:

- practising sitting meditation;
- practising standing up meditation;
- practising lying down meditation;
- practising walking meditation;
- and practising informal meditations like eating, doing the dishes and having a mindful bath.

Once you have built a mindfulness practice (and attending one of the eight-week courses can help you do this), you will also be able to bring into your day simple little breathing spaces like the three-minute dignities. You will be able to bring dignity to the stressful moments themselves and use your mindfulness directly, in the moment, almost like a super power.

But crucially, you just need to practise, whatever it is you're practising. So whether it's sitting, or standing, or reaching up for a tin of baked beans, you need to practise at it. It's difficult. But it's well worth it if you want to be well.

Building your mindfulness practice as a whole means you can find the spaciousness you need to address your relationship with stress, which is the crucial thing. Mindfulness helps you pause before you decide what to do next.

You can bring your mindfulness practice into your everyday life as Lorraine has

Hello, Philip here. It's over to Lorraine for the rest of this chapter but I thought I would poke my head in here and check how you're doing. How *are* you doing? It might just be the right time to jot down some words that represent how you're doing in this moment. Do a three-minute dignity and let the words that describe this moment come forward.

In this next section, Lorraine's going to give you a personal account of her own mindfulness practice and how she's used it for all kinds of stress, including a busy workload, a full-on family life, a medical condition, grief, and emotions like envy. During the ride, she will go deeper with a few of these ideas we've been talking about, to show how your mindfulness can be a great ally of your stressfulness. The key here, of course, is the *fullness*, your hidden fullness: finding the fullness that's already here, that's already with you.

So the invitation here is to think how you can bring some of this stuff into your own relationship with stress, so that you can start to build your own mindfulness practice. Don't forget, it's difficult to be anxious when you're curious.

Over to Lorraine with a personal account of using mindfulness for stress

On a practical level I meditate almost every morning for an average of 30 minutes. I'm lucky in that whether I intend to or not I am an early riser. I used to see this as a bit of an irritant, but these days the gift of time to fine tune myself into a mindfulness mode before tackling the demands of the day is much appreciated.

I do a full practice in the morning before work and I scatter little practices – like our three-minute dignities – throughout the day. Mostly I remember to try and eat mindfully as I munch the last mindful mouthful. I try and remember my mindfulness practice when I am walking the dogs or driving, when I have the opportunity to really stop and look at the surroundings and the conditions of the day. Traffic lights are a great opportunity to remember to breathe.

Eat a strawberry mindfully

Or a raisin, or a grape, or a curry. Take your piece of food – or your forkful – and slowly, gently, invite it into your frame of awareness. Approach it with the same civility and gentleness you might approach a deer in the woods.

Hold your strawberry (or whatever it is) up to the light. Are any bits of it translucent? Hold it in your palm, feel its own little gravitational pull tugging at your palm, and weigh it with kindness and non-judgement. Hold the strawberry between your fingers. Feel its sides with your fingers. Put the strawberry to your ear and listen to it. What sounds do strawberries make? Hold it up to your nose and smell it. Leave it close to your philtrum and roll it gently around your mouth.

Feel the strawberry get closer to your mouth. Feel it touch your lips – your top and bottom lips – and allow it to softly enter your mouth, but only very slowly. Let it rest halfway between the outside world and your mouth for as long as feels possible for you in this moment. When you let it fall into your mouth, do so with a gentle slowness that allows you to fully feel the strawberry now on your tongue, inside your mouth. Let it rest inside your mouth without biting down on it.

Then, gradually, bring your teeth to the strawberry and bite into it, again very slowly. Perhaps a little sinks down inside you straight away, leaving the rest of your strawberry in your mouth? Notice your strawberry disintegrate inside your wholeness; notice it becoming a part of you. Can you feel it make its way down your alimentary canal, even? When it has entirely left your mouth, how does your mouth feel now, in its absence? How do you feel, as a whole, that has borne witness to the natural order of things? What is your relationship with eating in this moment?

I use mindfulness breathing techniques when I feel anxious and afraid

Often I just straighten my posture to feel more in touch with my mountain-like qualities, tuning into the breath or breathing in to a count of 7 and out to 11, using the following exercise, which we loved so much (it's from Chris Cullen and Richard Burnett's Mindfulness in Schools programme) we had to share it with you.

Practise breathing whilst counting to 7 and 11

You can do this anywhere, whether it's your formal meditation practice or part of your everyday informal practice.

Settle into your position and simply, when you are ready, count to 7 on the in-breath. Notice the silence and the gap before the out-breath; and then count to 11 on the out-breath. Do this for as long as feels comfortable to you. If you can't reach either number, don't worry one bit, but generally you will find your out-breath is longer than your in-breath.

With practices like this, we really are making friends with ourselves and putting the welcome mat out to our experience of our breathing.

In the past I've had a terrible tendency to interpret events in a threatening or neurotic way

And I found that my mood changed for the worse or that my thoughts moved into a chaotic negative spiral as a result. Mindfulness has really helped me to temper this tendency and unpick the pattern of reaction, without even knowing the truth. Now, when I jump to a conclusion, I try to pause, and breathe, and just see if my thoughts are facts or just assumptions.

Realizing I can watch my thoughts and interrupt what I previously saw as a destructive, unleashed force has been revolutionary for me. I've realized I don't have to answer thoughts back. Even choosing not to follow the compelling pull of some thought or other has been transforming.

By going towards my feelings, I have gained the courage to face things and improve my ability to regulate myself

I still feel, but I am no longer afraid of my feelings. I used to feel bad for my thoughts, but now that I recognize my thoughts as neural firings, I know it is just my mind processing information it has gleaned, not signs of a bad character. The only responsibility I can take in this is whether or not I choose to feed my thoughts and what I do with them.

Mindfulness has been integrated into my life in a companionable way

My inner voice is being transformed. I do not say *has been transformed* because I am just a human being aspiring to live a more peaceful,

Reflect on how you might bring mindfulness into your own life

We appreciate there is a lot to learn still, and more importantly lots to practise, but even at this stage you can begin to wonder how you might bring mindfulness techniques into your own life in a way that is companionable. You've had a try of the main dignities – sitting, standing, lying down and walking – and you've also seen how much you can bring mindfulness practice into your everyday life – with everything from doing a three-minute dignity to washing the dishes mindfully and eating a mindful meal once a week. Jot down a few ways you might invite yourself to commit to being more mindful, particularly when it comes to stress, and your relationship with your stress. It doesn't matter if you can't commit to these things, they're just aspirations at the moment. Studies have shown, though, that writing things like this down – things that relate to values and the stuff you really care about – can help tremendously in enabling you to create a more meaningful life for yourself.

happier life. It has turned me into a kinder, wiser, more accepting friend than the old critical, threatened voice. It has helped me move towards believing the best of me, not the worst.

I have what could be described as very active mirror neurons

I pick up fear and anxiety from almost anywhere, and the reverse side of this is that I am also very empathic. Here's an example or two: the difficulty arises if I see blood on the screen or I am exposed to something tense; my body will react as if I am bleeding or being chased. As you can imagine, this is quite limiting. I can spend a considerable amount of time feeling the reactions of the stress response without them even being mine. In the past I would go straight into my mind to make sense of these feelings, fabricating or finding a reason why I should feel threatened. What a waste of energy and damaging adrenalin in my system!

Mindfulness has helped me with my stress factors

For most of my adult life, I have had a minor medical condition which means that I regularly have samples of blood taken. Objectively, I know this does not hurt (certainly not as much as plucking my eyebrows, which I do to myself voluntarily). However, for over 35 years I have always carried a bottle of Lucozade with me to the nephrologist in case I faint. I often have fainted, especially seeing blood in containers around me. When I explored this mindfully, I realized I was afraid of the *fear* I felt and not the thing itself. Now when I go into the room to have blood taken, I prepare myself by standing or sitting upright and doing some conscious breathing. I bring my awareness to the breath and notice the thoughts as they enter my mind, thoughts that have in them the sting of fear or doubt, and I let them pass. I might replace the thought

'Oh, I'm going to be sick!'

with

'I'm going to have a lovely drink when I'm finished.'

So I open myself up and walk out of my rigid thinking

If I'm doing well, I might even move beyond my own fear to being interested in the nephrologist and finding the opportunity for connection. Often when I tune into my body I recognize a heaviness in my chest and a clenching in my stomach, which I can either allow to intensify or notice and breathe through and soften. While I sit there I either keep my focus on my breath and feel grateful that I have had a moment to do a practice, or I get lost in the conversation and before I know it I am on my way to the coffee shop. I've stopped making a visit to the hospital automatically mean 'This is going to be stressful.'

Make mindful enquiries into your stress factors

Perhaps you could identify a situation in your life when you sometimes feel stressed. Maybe it's when you start to write something, or when you're in a traffic jam, or going to the dentist. Think of something a bit like my own trip to the nephrologist.

When you bring such a situation to mind, can you feel your body already starting to react? Maybe there's a tension in your shoulders or neck, a clenching of your jaw? So, let's pause right there and do a three-minute dignity.

Practise this briefly before holding a stressful moment in your attention. We will experiment with it at the mindfulness workbench. It's a very familiar part of mindfulness and involves lots of questions. At some level, mindfulness is all about enquiry.

Tune into the mindfulness station

Our attitude here is to be curious, not judgemental, for the next few moments. We are going to be kind and patient with ourselves.

Notice your posture as you hold your moment of stress in your awareness. Are you slouching? Are you standing stiffly to attention? Is it possible instead to move to the mountain position, to have a posture that is alert but not hyper-alert?

For a few moments, try connecting to the breath and gently steadying yourself. If you have problems with breathing or bringing attention to the breath – perhaps it makes you a bit panicky in itself, especially if you suffer from asthma – take your focused attention to your feet, the sensation of your feet in your shoes or the feeling of being held by the ground, tuning into your toes and then the soles and heels of your feet.

Here we bring the kind but firm attitude to invading thoughts. As best you can, bring yourself back to the breath or your feet. What's actually happening in the body? Let's be really interested. Let's not just say we're stressed but look at how it shows up. Is it in the shoulders? If it is, is it tight, heavy, rigid? Or can you feel your heartbeat in your stomach?

Kindly, let's see what happens if we turn to the symptoms themselves and not fight what we think they mean. Remember: it's hard to be anxious at the same time as being really curious. We could breathe into the areas of tightness, softening on the out-breath.

What's going on with your thoughts? Could we notice what they are saying? Perhaps it's something like: 'Why do I always get stuck in traffic', or, 'I am always sick at the dentist's', or, 'I am so scared', or 'I am so frustrated'.

Warmly, perhaps we could respond to these thoughts by simply pausing and observing them. So we're not answering them back, but just letting them pass, because they are filling us with propaganda that is not true – and even if it feels true we can still let them go.

How are you feeling emotionally? Even if you are feeling a bit stressed, it doesn't mean you can't move through it. So just breathe and steady yourself; keep counting the breath or observing your feet as you sit in the dentist's chair or wait for the traffic to clear. You might even notice the lovely cloud formation through the car windows or the interesting picture on the dentist's ceiling. The practice can help you pick up body signals more quickly rather than turning to automatic assumptions.

When you feel sensations of stress arising, adjust your posture so that you stand or sit in a more mountain-like way. Then try to be curious rather than reactive to your body. In doing this, you disconnect slightly from the power of those sensations.

This kind of enquiry is at the heart of mindfulness: how do you feel about it? Are you willing to make such enquiries yourself into your body and your experience of your stress factors?

This is very powerful stuff. You're effectively taking charge. It's none other than a radical act of potentially loving and learning from each and every moment.

Busy? Perfect. This is a great time to get mindful

I might tell myself I am going to slow down and live at a calmer pace, but my economic reality and my greed to have a go at everything means that there are very often times in my life when my work schedule is enormously busy. I do a lot of teaching and training, and at times it's a little scary if I look at the picture ahead of me. Perhaps I don't have a full day off for three weeks, or perhaps I have a whole group of things to prepare and carry out at the same time. As a result, I can become overwhelmed and a bit mentally paralysed by the prospect of it all. I might then come down with a load of physical ailments, with sleepless nights to add to the fun.

During these frantic periods of my life I used to become very stressed, which would manifest in me being irritable and bad tempered with my family and friends, tearful, unable to think properly. I would become very disorganized and forgetful and full of self-loathing, as I would tell myself it was All My Fault. I would ruin everything by feeling I was 'so stupid to allow this to happen again'. I would give up things that nourished me, thinking I didn't have the time to meditate or relax.

Mindfulness has helped me to realize that I can manage these times

Mindfulness is not only accessible in calm, quiet times but through all life's conditions. We can learn to use the practices we have built up to recognize how the stress machine works and become aware that we can make even the most chaotic times more manageable. If we use mindful moments strategically, they offer an amazing opportunity for practice.

Stop making busy automatically mean unhappy and stressed

It's easy to do, right? Instead of waiting for the stress to pass so that your life can begin, realize – with real eyes – that this stressful moment is in fact entirely your life. The moments of intense work can be some of the most meaningful and enjoyable, the connections you make some of the deepest. When they are clustered together, it is easy to forget to see and appreciate this.

Mindfulness helps you live each moment with more presence and take time to notice and drink in the pleasure

I used to feel so guilty about being away from my family when I was busy that I would let the stress of constantly preparing to go away stop me from being truly present. As a result, the times I did have with my family would be full of arguments and tensions. Now I try to live the moments without letting my thoughts carry me off to the next piece of work, and without worries of 'what if' and 'if only' filling my head. Now I am much better at being fully with my family. When I am there, time feels so much richer and I am no longer constantly trying to climb out of the deficit of how I think it ought to be and into the loveliness of how it is. That's so nice, let's say it again. With mindfulness, we can . . .

Climb out of the deficit of *how we think it ought to be*, into the loveliness of *how it is*

I realize that in times of busyness I need to resource myself with more meditation and nourishing activities, not fewer. The meditation sets me up for the day, helps me to concentrate and focus so I get more done and forget less. It reminds me to notice beauty, so I am carried along with a sense of satisfaction, not resentment, and it helps me manage moments of potential stress and stop them escalating.

Since I began practising mindfulness my workload has increased and my life has become more demanding

We have moved house and city, I have had surgery twice, and my mother died after going through a gruelling illness. Three of these major life events happened at the same time. The gift of mindfulness helped me to be present to all. Time seemed to grow. The only times I felt really out of balance were when my practice declined. I do not think I would have been able to cope with all the pressures without it. And although those times were demanding and very sad, I have been able to cultivate a sense of happiness and gratitude I did not have before.

Make mindfulness with your busyness

So let's move into the being mode for a few moments, away from the constant doing mode where we're letting our lives run past us while we think or plan something else. Being is the attitudinal foundation we need to employ for this task. Accepting and letting be means we allow our life to unfold as it is rather than assuming how it is going to be. Here we take on beginner's mind. We don't need to know or remember the future or the past, here in the present.

Be aware of what you are making everything mean

Are you equating busyness with stress or unhappiness? Does this equation represent the absolute truth? Can you start the day by either following your breath for just a few moments or listening to a brief guided body scan, not by automatically going into list mode? You could even put stickers on your phone, car or kettle to remind you to Stop and Take a Mindful Pause, or maybe set a timer on your phone to go off a few times a day to remind you that

You are alive.

When you feel a sensation of being overwhelmed or the beginnings of the stress response:

- Can you do a three-minute dignity?
- Can you bring your awareness to your thoughts?
- Can you notice if your thoughts are taking you away from where you are?
- Can you become mountain-like and let your thoughts pass?
- Can you bring to your awareness some of the things you love about your life right now?
- Can you fall in love with your life just that little bit more?
- Can you avoid getting caught up in how you think things ought to be and just be with things as they are?
- Can you be that accepting?

Another stress factor in my life is that I sometimes compare myself to others

This means, I am somewhat ashamed to admit, that sometimes in the past I have been consumed with envy, or at least I haven't always wanted the best for my friends or colleagues. This has often been very uncomfortable for me to cope with, something I felt deeply ashamed of. So I would suppress it, keeping myself awake at night trying to control it with my thoughts, comparing myself to other people, judging myself, feeling threatened as if other people's good luck would somehow mean my bad luck, making their success more about me and my inadequacies than about them. I longed to be able to 'rejoice in their merits', as the Buddhists would say. And then I would stay awake worrying about being inauthentic or mean.

Mindfulness has helped me take the stress out of this in many ways

Maybe the greatest help for me here was the attitude of compassion to myself, realizing that whatever I was feeling was OK because that was how I felt. Accepting this and not judging it or striving to make it different really allowed me to own those feelings and not push them away. With mindfulness we can bring to mind a difficulty and go towards it with curiosity and kindness. The important thing here is that we do not go into the story or all the accompanying thoughts, but we notice how it turns up in the body and what happens to those feelings if we gently and kindly give them our attention.

I realized I had a whole mixture of feelings and emotions, tightness in the chest and shoulders, a sinking knotted feeling in my jaw and a tight band across my head. My thoughts were invasive, judgemental, critical and hard to keep at bay. My emotions were a caustic mixture of fear, inadequacy and shame, leaving me with a deep sense of being unworthy and unloveable.

This all arrived through excruciating physical sensations I would try and avoid through impulses and habits like eating chocolate and buying clothes. With practice I became able to bring compassion to myself and not get caught up in the story and the thoughts; like magic, often the symptoms would disappear. When the thoughts occurred at night, I would often feed them by trying to think my way through them, but this would only make them grow.

Mindfulness has taught me that for the most part you cannot heal emotional distress with thoughts. Instead I just come to the body scan of breathing with love and compassion, not needing it to be other than it is. Then, cradled in my own compassion, I will get myself to sleep by realizing it makes me feel so much more at ease and happy when I let go of control and really feel, for example, the happiness of my friend's success. I feel as if I am in my own skin again. I am not saying that I no longer get feelings of jealousy, but when they arise within me I can go up close and release the stronghold and it is a lovely, liberating, joyous feeling to really feel pleased for a friend. I have also realized what high expectations I have of myself. I have realized it is good to be ordinary and human and that I can still be worthy of love.

Here we need compassion, non-judgement, curiosity and patience

Perhaps next time you feel the twinge or sting of an unpleasant thought, stop and go into the mountain and breathe, or focus on your feet – whatever grounds and centres you – and where possible give yourself the time to attend to yourself kindly. This does not mean ruminating on the story and intensifying the mood by analysing your thoughts; it does mean giving yourself room to take a look at the sensations and thoughts evoked by the mood.

My most stressful time recently was when I went through a period of low mood

It only lasted a couple of weeks but I felt exhausted and unhappy. I felt I was a fraud in that I had been teaching mindfulness but could not manage my own moods. I had rigid thoughts and a fixed goal. My inner sentence went something like 'Doing mindfulness means that I should never feel low.' This caused me such stress and disappointment and only increased my negative spiral of thoughts, feelings and mood.

Fortunately, I have a very wise mindfulness teacher who was quickly able to identify that I was committing a simple mindfulness mistake:

I wanted things to be different.

I was not accepting my condition; instead I was striving to fix it. As soon as I was able to see this I stopped my thoughts spiralling down. I turned to myself with compassion and beginner's mind. I allowed

Get yourself a mindfulness teacher

This book is written by a mindfulness teacher (Lorraine) and one of her students (Philip). The relationship between teacher and student is really important, not only in mindfulness but across all art forms and apprenticeships. We can't recommend highly enough that you find your own real-life mindfulness teacher. Mindfulness is very much a lived experience and though books are helpful, nothing replicates the one-to-one and group experiences of the eight-week mindfulness course. Find your nearest course at <www.bemindful.co.uk> and go fishing for your teacher. The teacher–student relationship can be a hugely rewarding paradigm where both of you can learn and expand your abilities to be open-hearted. Both of us, Lorraine and Philip, have learnt loads from each other. When it comes to mindfulness, the teacher is really our breath, our heartbeats, our stillness, our silence. We are all of us students of the present moment.

myself to be held in the larger container of mindfulness and returned to the warming ritual of listening. Most of all, I rested: the mood was born of exhaustion and the beginnings of an infection, but I had made it mean something completely different. I was tired and needed nourishment and small useful things instead of pushing myself by analysing and forcing.

With mindfulness we begin to recognize the early warning signs of negative moods, anxiety or depression

We attempt to develop the habit of stopping and breathing, taking the temperature of our sensations, thoughts and feelings. Very often at these times we need to support ourselves or motivate ourselves to act, before the negative mood spiral or habit sets in. So after we do a dignity, we do something or plan to do something nourishing or something to help us feel motivated. If we are in a low mood, it's important to remember that it's no use waiting to be motivated before we do something. We need to do a little action first to create motivation. It can be something that gives us a sense of agency, like watering a plant, answering one email or chopping one vegetable instead of reaching for the biscuit barrel.

If times are tough, bring awareness to your coping strategy

In preparation for the difficult times, as well as keeping up the practice, we also need to know our repertoire of automatic coping mechanisms. Our impulses at these times can be helpful, but more often than not they backfire on us. It might be worthwhile for you just to think of how you automatically, habitually release or avoid your feelings. How do you avoid your feelings? Is it by:

- sleeping
- shouting
- cleaning
- drinking alcohol

- eating chocolate
- watching TV
- crying
- ruminating?

Although some of these have short-term gains, avoiding your negative feelings hardly ever works. The habits can turn into addictions, all trying to run away from a feeling.

We can practise using a pause filled with dignity – a breathing space where we can stop, centre ourselves and review. As before:

- shift your posture;
- bring your focus of attention to your breathing;
- take a temperature gauge of your feelings, sensations and thoughts, observing them so you step outside them;
- and then see what you need to do.

We trust that this too will pass

I spent most of my life believing I was stuck with an anxious mind and a sensitive body. I believed this was a permanent temperamental bias and the last 40 years of my life have been a journey of working out how to manage it, so I could have some adventure.

When I was 16 and hospitalized for the first time with a severe kidney infection, I was put on tranquillizers for symptoms of anxiety and depression (I would call it a touch of existential angst now). I was warned by the medical profession not to be too ambitious or stray too far, or else I would be dead by the time I was 40. Then followed 30 years of journeying, personally and professionally, through psychology and different strands of spirituality into ways to manage my limitations and develop resilience. It wasn't until I discovered mindfulness-based stress reduction that I saw everything I had been following come together, saw the evidence of research and neuroscience that I could, through mindfulness, systematically manage my anxieties and cultivate the means to change my temperamental bias.

I discovered that the brain is plastic and that continued practice can change its very structure.

With mindfulness, you create the freedom to see the world the way it is, to love every single moment

With this simple practice, it is possible to choose the best response to any situation and escape the cage of conditioned reactions. My previous limiting propaganda of thoughts about myself were not the absolute truth. Although I am very much at the beginning of this journey, mindfulness has given me the tools to take some control in my life. It has given me the hope that I can move towards greater and greater peace of mind and contentment.

Mindfulness practice really does magnify the lens of awareness and appreciation of the beauty around you

Even in the starkest of places, it has given me the wondrous gift of noticing and finding delight in the smallest things. I can't say I always act upon it, but I am more appreciative of my relationships and endeavour always to be more mindful.

When it is working, my mindfulness enables me to be less reactive and more productive in my responses to things. Strangely, this often helps me to get the things I need and the responses I want far more than the old reactive patterns.

If it's of interest, this is possible for you too

Did you know that? Yes, it is possible through mindfulness to rewrite your relationship with stress, and say yes, yes, yes to your stress as a meaningful part of your much bigger life.

5

Loving every moment

So here we are, at the other end of the book

What have we learnt?

- We are lovely, whoever we are, because we each have a beautiful stillness at our centre.
- Stress probably isn't what we thought it was.
- Stress can be good, stress can be bad, stress can be useful, stress can be debilitating.
- Mindfulness is a practice that helps us explore our stress. Mindfulness is a great ally of stressfulness.
- There is no such thing as stress as such. There are simply stress factors and stress responses. We can bring mindfulness to both.
- It's stressful because you care about it. That's why it's stressful. When it's stressful and you don't care about it, mindfulness can help you enquire into what is going on for you. Perhaps it's something else?
- We can practise mindfulness to help us explore our relationship with stress. Working on our stress mindset as a whole can help us shift. When we shift, new things happen, new possibilities open up.
- We can change our relationship to stress. Our brains are plastic, we can practise getting better at observing our thoughts as thoughts and not following them. We can take control of our meaning making.

- We can use all sorts of mindfulness practices as part of our ongoing experiment with stress. We can sit, stand, move, walk or eat mindfully, and we can use the brief three-minute dignity practice in any moment, particularly in stressful ones, to give us space and spaciousness and the ability to choose how to respond, not react.
- To any stress factor, with mindfulness we can gently ask of our stress response system: do I need to run away, freeze, fight, comply, fly, learn or grow, or perhaps a mixture of them? We can ask, 'What do I need in this moment?'
- Mindfulness can help us love every moment, not because it's unashamedly positive as a technique or practice – it's not at all – but because it suggests that each moment is rich in meaningful potential, even (and especially) the difficult, stressful ones.
- Mindfulness is particularly good for experiencing the joys of life – like eating your favourite ice cream – and it is particularly good for experiencing the difficulties of life – like being confronted with a stress factor.

Have a really slow, mindful bath

Baths are great for practising mindfulness of stress. Allow yourself 35–40 minutes for a really lovely, slow, mindful bath. Let yourself be slow and light and full of ease, as you turn on the bath taps, pour your favourite bath bubbles in, and prepare yourself to sink into the warm and wet loveliness. Attend to how you move in the bath, do a bath body scan – the water can help you attend to parts of your body you might not ordinarily feel so easily! Be mindful of the water on your skin, compare it to how the air normally feels. How is the waterscape different? Ask yourself mindful questions, as we practised earlier, to help you make enquiries into your lived experience. And as you leave the experience of the bath, prepare yourself by checking in: how does it feel to let go of this bath? Make sure you have the cleanest, loveliest, softest pyjamas to wear after your mindfulness bath.

Mindfulness simply lets you turn up to the present moment

It's great for dealing with stress, but it's great for dealing with anything that's occurring to you in your present moment. The hard part is turning up to your present moment, really turning up to what is happening here and now. It's very easy to talk about, but difficult to experience. So use the practices – the sitting, the standing, the lying down and walking meditations – as ways into your present moment. Only then, when you have turned up, can you begin to attend to the stress factor of the moment. In a way, the mindfulness bit is pre-stress. It's outside the stress. It's what you need to practise to get to the stress. Without mindfulness, you might be destined to never see what really is in this moment, what really is the cause of the stress you are experiencing.

In a way, mindfulness slows you down so that you can begin to see again

It's a bit like on TV, when they use slow motion. When you practise mindfulness, you slow yourself down and in doing so, you open up a spaciousness that is always there, but that just needs revealing.

So point the mindfulness remote control at yourself and press Pause

With the spaciousness, you can do so much:

- You can enjoy the experience you are experiencing even more, or you can ready yourself to learn more from the experience.
- You can bear witness to your reactions in the moment.
- You can inhabit the gap between a stress factor and your stress response, akin to the gap between the in-breath and the out-breath.
- You can smell, taste, touch, feel the moment in its richness, in its simplicity and plainness, and in its textured complexity.

- You can get ready to carry forward your great, positive self – the 'better angels of our nature', as Abraham Lincoln said – and prepare to make positive steps in your life that lead to change and possibility and discovery.

Make time for a day of mindfulness

You don't have to just use mindfulness in moments of stress, and mindfulness is certainly not designed only for stress. You can carve out time in your busy diary for mindfulness, whole days of mindfulness if you like. It's a lovely thing to do, to make yourself a mindfulness day retreat in your own home. Make sure you find a time when you won't be disturbed. If you have kids, go out of your way to get a babysitter; you're important and it's important that you find this time for yourself. When you give yourself a mindfulness retreat, you can practise the main dignities – sitting, standing, lying down and walking – alongside informal mindfulness exercises like mindful eating, doing the dishes mindfully and having a mindful bath. You can write in your journal about recent stresses and strains and how you have responded to them, how your mindfulness practice has helped (or not, if that is also true). You can listen to music mindfully, or go for a walk outside and enjoy the simplicity of leaves and light. If you have been sharing this work with a friend, you could even do the mindfulness retreat as a pair, and have mindful dialogue between stretches of gorgeous silence.

It is because of this spaciousness opened up by mindfulness that you can love every moment

Every moment – even the so-called worst, most stressful moments – are up for being loveable. Because you are becoming more in control of your life, because you are using mindfulness to help you take the lead when it comes to stress response, you are making it possible to love every moment. When we love every moment, we are leading our lives. We are living our lives authentically.

With mindful spaciousness, we don't get rid of stress, but we might get to enjoy our stress

We shift from 'Oh, I have to do the dishes' to 'Oooh, I get to do the dishes'. We put the fullness back into stressfulness. We begin to flirt with our stress, to dance with it, we even begin to fall in love with our stress. Our stress, rather than being something we want to delete from our lives, becomes one of the most interesting things about us. We begin to suggest that our stress is our charm. We get better at being stressed, rather than better at getting rid of our stress. Mindfulness of stress as a strategy is a strategy of friendship with ourselves. We befriend our stress, we write letters to our stress. We breathe, we stand in our tall stillness, and we put our hands out as an offering to our stress. To approach our stress with mindfulness – to approach it like the deer in the woods it is – is to embrace our stress as an integral part of our life, as important – as a conveyor of meaning – as the best of our dreams, wishes, intentions and passions. It is to realize that stress is more.

And we've not just made this up, of course

Mindfulness is 2,500 years old, and probably older, and though connected with religious traditions like Buddhism, it is a secular practice supported by tons of contemporary scientific research. For example in the UK, mindfulness is recommended by NICE, the government's National Institute for Health and Care Excellence. And there's growing evidence that mindfulness can be used in all kinds of settings, like:

- schools and universities
- prisons
- workplaces
- hospitals and pregnancy units.

We've not had the time or space to go into the research, but we point to some at the end, in case you're interested, which is good if you are.

When we approach our stress mindfully, we walk in a landscape of possibility

That is our main wish for you: to walk in a landscape of possibility. When you approach life with mindfulness, you find the space you need to walk in possibility, in gratitude and in beauty. And walking in possibility, in gratitude, in beauty means new openings, new shift-ings, new patterns of being. When we shift ourselves in this way, we shift our whole ecology, our whole environment – we become kinder, softer, more gentle, more willing. It is no small thing to say that we benefit the entire universe with this work of approaching our stress with mindfulness.

There's something lovely about you

We said so at the start, and we'll say it again. There's something lovely about you. And it's something to do with your stillness, your breathing, your simply being here, holding this book. It's what Christopher Isherwood in his amazing book about yoga, *My Guru and his Disciple*, called 'this thing', the indescribable experience of being in the now.

You and your stress are a beautiful part of the world. Even in this brief moment, this brief book, you will have softened your gaze towards your stress.

So take this moment, as we come to a close, to do a three-minute dignity:

- Gently stop in this moment, and notice your breathing.
- Look around you, and then bring your gaze inwards and look throughout your body, feeling the contact with the earth in this moment.
- Then listen, to sounds outside, but also to the sounds inside your body, and the sounds of thinking, that you are invited to just observe, without following.

And then, once you are centred in this way, drop this sentence into your awareness and this time, come to it afresh, anew, with beginner's mind and a non-judgemental attitude:

There's something lovely about me.

How does that feel now? Do you trust the sentence now? How patient can you be with it, as it drops slowly through you like a pebble in a stream? Can you let it just be, this sentence that's offering you a hug in this moment, without striving with it, without trying to get anywhere? Can you accept its meaning, and by accepting, let it go? And now, how does that feel, letting this sentence that says you're lovely go? How does it feel just to be here in the plainness and simplicity of your lived experience?

Because this too will pass

With mindfulness, we stand tall, like a mountain, and watch all these things – all our stresses, all our joys – go up in the sky, rising like balloons, before they vanish into the distance, on the horizon. They leave us breathing, with more than a half-smile, back down on planet Earth, in our neighbourhood, on our street, standing on the welcome mat at our front door.

And so we begin again, freed in the spacious gap we have created for ourselves. And we start to take our next steps into the landscape of what's possible and meaningful and beautiful in our lives, knowing it's tricky to be anxious if we're curious.

And as we walk, we hold hands with ourselves, and with our stresses and our strains, which are part of our lives, only now our lives are bigger. We know that, with mindfulness, you don't necessarily shrink stress, but you do enlarge the life around it.

May you be well, adventurer

As we sign off, as we notice that the number of pages available to us is running out, we want to thank you for getting this far and for coming along with us on our journey.

In many ways this book is a right old mish-mash – sometimes science, sometimes wonder, sometimes instruction, sometimes personal anecdote – but throughout it's been a joy to write, a real collaboration between friends, between teacher and student, student and teacher, and we've loved you being here, co-creating these words by reading them. It's felt like we've been whispering some ideas in your gorgeous head. Thank you for that.

It's time for you to go now, too, though, and so suffice to say: may you go very well indeed. Good luck with all that you do with the ideas we've laid out for you here, like clothes laid out on a bed. Choose what works for you, sign up for a mindfulness course if possible, and keep in touch with your breathing, as we will keep in touch with ours. Thank you for being here. Thank you for all the good work you are doing and about to do as you examine lived experience from the big toes up. Cheers from us. Cheers and cheerio.

Further reading

Below we've listed some books you might want to have a look at as you develop your mindfulness practice. As we've said, attending one of the eight-week courses can be really helpful; find your nearest one, including plenty of evidence and research that backs up why mindfulness is so effective, at <http://bemindful.co.uk>, and may you be well, safe and protected, happy and whole, to whatever degree is possible, as you embark on your mindfulness journey.

Christopher Germer, *The Mindful Path to Self-Compassion* (New York: The Guilford Press, 2009)

Jon Kabat-Zinn, *Full Catastrophe Living* (London: Piatkus, 2001)

Jon Kabat-Zinn, *Wherever You Go, There You Are* (London: Piatkus, 2004)

Jon Kabat-Zinn, *Coming To Our Senses* (London: Piatkus, 2005)

David McCown and Marc S. Micozzi, *New World Mindfulness* (Randolph, Vermont: Healing Arts Press, 2012)

Kelly McGonigal, *The Upside of Stress* (London: Vermilion, 2015)

Thich Nhat Hanh, *The Miracle of Mindfulness* (London: Rider, 2008)